Walking with a Shadow

Walking with a Shadow

Surviving Childhood Leukemia

NANCI A. SULLIVAN

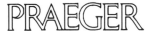 Westport, Connecticut
London

Library of Congress Cataloging-in-Publication Data

Sullivan, Nanci A., 1957–
    Walking with a shadow : surviving childhood leukemia / Nanci A. Sullivan.
        p. cm.
    Includes bibliographical references and index.
    ISBN 0-275-95814-0 (alk. paper)
    1. Leukemia in children.   2. Leukemia in children—Case studies.   I. Title.
RJ416.L4S84   2004
362.19'89299419'0092—dc22   2004045938
    [B]

British Library Cataloguing in Publication Data is available.

Library of Congress Catalog Card Number: 2004045938
ISBN: 0-275-95814-0

First published in 2004

Praeger Publishers, 88 Post Road West, Westport, CT 06881
An imprint of Greenwood Publishing Group, Inc.
www.praeger.com

Printed in the United States of America

The paper used in this book complies with the
Permanent Paper Standard issued by the National
Information Standards Organization (Z39.48-1984).

10 9 8 7 6 5 4 3 2 1

Children with cancer are more than children seeking to live.
They are a symbol of hope and possibility.

—John J. Spinetta, *Living with Childhood Cancer*

What the caterpillar sees as the tragedy of death,
the butterfly sees as the miracle of birth.

—John Marks Templeton

This literary accomplishment is dedicated to those who participated as part of my research for my dissertation and for the field-initiated grant. Without these incredible human beings who were willing to retell their stories of childhood cancer so that future children could benefit from their experiences, this book would not have existed. They were the "wind beneath my wings" that kept me persevering during the most difficult times of writing this book. Their life stories deserve to be told to all who are willing to listen and learn.

This book is also dedicated to all children who must, without choice, face the challenges of the childhood cancer experience—diagnosis, treatment, long-term survival, and quite possibly death. These children are experiencing at a young age great adversity but learning wisdom and an appreciation beyond their years of the gift of life. They are the true heroes and the shining stars of this earthly world.

To my mentor, colleague, and friend, Dr. Mary Ravita, who is living with cancer and fighting a brave, gallant battle against it. I am sure with her immense determination and positiveness she will prevail. She is a role model to all of us in facing one of life's greatest challenges with grace and dignity.

Lastly, my book is also dedicated to family and friends who lost an arduous battle against cancer but who quietly taught me by example the true meaning of life, courage, and faith. These individuals will never be forgotten, for their memories are etched in my mind forever and they are always only a breath away.

Ferne Stella McClaskey Shonek, paternal grandmother, February 15, 1969
Dorothy Johnston, neighbor and friend, September 12, 1995
Colleen Petrisko, neighbor and friend, February 26, 1996
Barbara Brokaw, neighbor and friend, January 25, 2000

Jayne Reda, colleague and friend, February 7, 2001
Joan Boston, neighbor and friend, October 28, 2001
Belinda Williamson Scalise, high school classmate and friend, December 8, 2002

Contents

PART ONE   SURVIVING

Foreword

To confront a person with his own shadow
is to show him his own light.

—Carl G. Jung

Childhood cancer is an unwanted reality in the lives of many children. While the number of children diagnosed is gradually increasing, the effectiveness of treatment protocols is increasing even more rapidly. Thus more and more of these children survive into young adulthood and beyond. Consequently, more individuals living with cancer, and more individuals who have survived cancer, are found in our families, our classrooms, and our places of employment. Almost 10,000 children in the United States are diagnosed with cancer each year. A teacher with a forty-year teaching career will have had, on average, four students who have been diagnosed with cancer. Very few of us will live our lives without encountering a childhood cancer survivor as a family member, a student, a friend, or a colleague. The increasing presence of surviving children and young adults calls for a greater level of understanding on the part of all of us. A book that would provide information about childhood cancer in a form that could be understood by nonmedical personnel would be welcomed by many of us.

Walking with a Shadow by Nanci Sullivan does much more than provide such needed information. Yes, the *facts* of childhood cancer—especially acute lymphoblastic leukemia, which until recently was the most common cancer of childhood—are presented in up-to-date and readily understood detail. But what really draws the reader into the world of childhood cancer are the stories of children living with and surviving the disease. The author recounts the stories of nine individuals, all diagnosed with acute lymphoblastic leukemia between the ages of five and seven, who are now between eighteen and thirty-four years of age. Dr. Sullivan's technique of heavily relying on the actual words of the participants to tell their stories brings to the reader a sense of engagement in the day-to-day life of someone living with cancer. The principals, now young adults, all have experienced years of struggling with cancer. The passage of time has provided each of them the opportunity to reflect on the presence of the "shadow" and each of them shares with us the private world of dealing with that "shadow." Readers will find similarities in the stories, but also differences—as one would expect from individuals coping with life-threatening conditions.

The recollections of the discomfort, pain, loneliness, and uncertainty of the cancer treatments experienced by the survivors provide insight and offer implications for such treatment. However, the aspect of childhood cancer that is most poignant is the fact that the disease, even as it is being vanquished by treatment protocols, extracts from the patient a lasting cost in learning difficulties. A majority of these young adults reported problems in attention and concentration, memory and mathematics difficulties, and reading comprehension problems. Extensive independent research has attributed such difficulties to the effects of the cancer treatment.

While the cancer survivors, in their own words, tell us their stories, we also hear glimpses of the stories of their parents and siblings. A diagnosis of cancer, after all, affects not only the subject individuals, but also their families. This is particularly true when the persons diagnosed are young children, as was the case with all the individuals here. We read that Patricia's parents did not tell her that she had cancer until she was seventeen. Elaine on the other hand doesn't remember a time when she didn't know, although her parents actually had taken two or three years to tell her. Readers cannot help but wonder about the anguish of parents who had to decide whether and how to tell a five to seven-year-old child that he or she had cancer.

The latter part of *Walking with a Shadow* puts the entire issue of childhood cancer into perspective for families and schools. From the survivor's stories, Dr. Sullivan has gleaned implications and recommendations to improve educational and psychosocial outcomes. Parents and teachers will welcome the specificity and practicality of this information. The chapter

"When a Child Dies" includes in its entirety a wonderful article on grief and death in the classroom—a topic rarely considered except in cases of violent death, as in school shootings. This chapter is essential reading for all teachers.

Walking with a Shadow concludes with a comprehensive list of resources for families, friends, teachers, and coworkers. Included are books, videos, television shows, and web sites that provide information and support.

In her epilogue, Dr. Sullivan asks "What greater impact can one have than to have survivors teach you the true meaning of life?" The stories recounted in her book can help all of us "learn from our journeys, trials, and tribulations so we are able through ourselves to give life lessons as gifts back to others." This book is a gift to all of us.

Nettie R. Bartel, Ph.D
Temple University
Philadelphia, PA
March 17, 2004

Preface

Be willing to accept the shadows that walk across the sun.

—Emmanuel

Cancer does not discriminate against age, gender, nationality, or geographic location. Children acquire cancer just as adults do. Acute lymphoblastic leukemia is second to brain tumors as the first most common form of childhood cancer. Cancer is the second leading cause of death in children under the age of 15 (accidents being the first).

However, there is reason for optimism. Children are surviving cancer in greater numbers than ever before. But with survival comes a new set of problems. Doctors, families, teachers, and survivors now need to be concerned about reintegration back into school and about the learning, psychosocial, and physiological problems that survivors encounter. Each year schools face increasing numbers of students who are entering school with chronic or even life-threatening medical illnesses. Educational personnel must continue to learn how to support these children in the school environment. Their support is critical to the physiological, psychosocial, and educational spirit of children experiencing and surviving cancer. A diagnosis of cancer is always unexpected particularly in children. All individuals who are part of the child's life become overwhelmed and disheartened. However, parents and educators need to remember that even though the child has cancer she or he still develops and grows physically, emotionally, and socially during the time of treatment and posttreatment.

In this book, we hear from long-term survivors of childhood acute lymphoblastic leukemia. Through the nine stories told by childhood cancer survivors who are now adults, we experience a snapshot of the impact that the cancer experience has on all aspects of a child's life. The stories contained in this book, challenging as they may seem, are stories of hope and survival. For many of the participants in this project, it was the first time anyone had asked them about their journey from diagnosis to treatment to cure to reintegration back into school and to adult lives. Several of these young people told me that the interview I conducted was the first time that they themselves actually went back in time and walked through the experience again. Many found the interview therapeutic or cathartic. I hope that the insights of these survivors will be of use to pediatric oncologists, psychologists, nurses, teachers, parents, and the other survivors of childhood cancer. I believe that the stories, common themes, and recommendations sections of this book will also be useful to those who work with children who have chronic and catastrophic illnesses other than childhood cancer.

We speak often in our society about heroes, mentors, and role models that have had a positive or life-altering affect on our lives. Children look up to adults such as sports figures or celebrities. I consider the individuals who told me their stories as heroes, mentors, and role models as well; they found great inner strength with purity and innocence to survive one of life's most devastating and painful traumas—cancer. Heroes know fear intimately, and yet they walk through life with uncommon quiet courage. Courage is not the absence of fear, but rather facing the fear and continuing to do what one needs to do to survive.

Teachers look at children and young adults as learners, but in this book children are the teachers. The stories contained herein display some of the greatest educational and life lessons to be learned. If there is one single purpose why we are on this earth, it is to help and support each other through our life lessons. When someone shares with us their experiences, they are teachers who are trying to say to us "I want you to know. I want you to see through my eyes. I want you to hear through my ears." When you read this book, I hope you experience their journeys, and their life lessons, and their exuberance of life, and that it causes you to pause and reflect on your own life.

This intriguing work came about unexpectedly for me. However, I have found that some of life's greatest treasures are found unexpectedly. As I was preparing for doctoral comprehensive examinations and researching various topics on the computer at the library, I came upon an article that described reading and math difficulties as well as psychosocial problems in school environments as posttreatment effects of surviving acute lymphoblastic leukemia. The article immediately sparked my interest, so I contacted its author, Raymond Mulhern, at St. Jude's Hospital in Nashville, Tennessee. He was gracious as well as generous. He talked to me at some length about his work on the relationship between cancer treatment and learning/emotional problems. Dr. Mulhern sent me all of his articles on this topic. After reading them, I tracked down at least 40 to 50 research studies written by pediatric oncologists and the like, and I discovered a few of the articles were about research being conducted in Pittsburgh, Pennsylvania, at Children's Hospital under the direction of Dr. Vincent Albo. I felt certain at this juncture that I could develop a study at the University of Pittsburgh by collaborating with professionals at Children's Hospital. I proceeded to formulate a dissertation on the educational and psychosocial sequelae of surviving acute lymphoblastic leukemia and its treatment regimes. But rather than doing another quantitative study, I decided to do a qualitative study, interviewing long-term survivors about their perceptions and reflections of their childhood cancer experience.

This book was an offshoot of my doctoral dissertation and a subsequent longitudinal study conducted by Naomi Zigmond, Debra Fulmer, and me funded by a grant from the U.S. Department of Education, Office of Special Education Programs. The title for the book emerged as I wrote the participants' stories of survival and completed my analysis of their experiences that they had shared with me. The young survivors in this book repeated numerous times that even though they had been cured of childhood cancer for many years, the experience clouded all parts of their lives, like a shadow. It was apparent to me that even though life was going well for them now, when the sun had come out again in their lives, the shadow of their survivor experience walks with them in their daily lives. They have struggled to accept the shadows just as they accept the sun in the journey of their lives.

Acknowledgments

It is the realization that we are loved that saves us when the
world around us crumbles.

—Melissa Kelly

This work literally would not have been possible without the courageous
and often challenging efforts of the young survivors who told their stories
of cancer survival with great hopes of helping other children who will
face this journey. They also wanted to provide insight to individuals who
work with children who are fighting and surviving cancer. Thank you to
Dr. Raymond Mulhern, St. Jude's Hospital, for planting the seeds of my
passionate interest, and to Dr. Vincent Albo, Children's Hospital of Pittsburgh, for providing his support in this endeavor, as well as offering access to lists of long-term survivors from the patient archives at Children's
Hospital. Without Dr. Albo, there would have been no stories. To Dr.
Naomi Zigmond, my adviser and friend, who believed in me when I did
not, for providing me autonomy to pursue this research, and a special
deep gratitude for her friendship, support, and expert editing skills. A
special thank you to Debbie Fulmer for being my second pair of hands,
eyes, and legs in the preparation and completion of this book. To Katie, a
graduate student, my gratitude for her help in preparing the bibliotherapy section of the book. Thanks also to Dave Matta for his assistance with
the editing and preparation of the text for submission to the publisher. To

Dr. Joseph M. Romanello, my thanks for his unwavering encouragement in my research and in this book. To Karen Scanlon, Suzanne Padeliadu, and Lea Kozminsky, who were my friends and doctoral cohorts and who challenged my intellect to its maximum potential so this book could be created. To Carol Holleran, a friend, who came into my life at just the right time to lift my spirits and help me enjoy the good things in life so I could complete this book. To Christina Simcic, a friend who has given me the gift of reflection and depth of soul to become a better person while listening and giving to others. She created the drawings for my book. To my family for loving me enough to let go of me so I could soar to pursue my dreams. To past teachers and mentors who supported me and believed in me at critical times in my life—Judy Fortunato, Allison Harris, and Mary Lucille Smith. Lastly, to Greenwood Publishing Group for being captivated by the stories of these remarkable individuals and for their encouragement to pursue this publication.

Prayer of a Writer

Lord of all things, whose wondrous gifts to man
Include the shining symbols known as words,
Grant that I may use their mighty power
Only for good. Help me to pass on
Small fragments of Your wisdom, truth, and love.
Teach me to touch the unseen, lonely heart
With laughter, or the quick release of tears.
Let me portray the courage that endures
Defiant in the face of pain or death;
The kindness and the gentleness of those
Who fight against the anger of the world;
The beauty hidden in the smallest things;
The mystery, the wonder of it all. . . .
Open my ears, my eyes; unlock my heart.
Speak through me, Lord, if it be Your will. Amen.

—Excerpt from
A Touch of Wonder
by Arthur Gordon

Introduction

Nothing in life is more exciting and rewarding than the
sudden flash of insight that leaves you a changed person—
not only changed, but changed for the better. Such
moments are rare, certainly, but they come to all of
us. Sometimes from a book, a sermon, a line of
poetry. Sometimes from a friend or a stranger. . . .

—Arthur Gordon, *A Touch of Wonder*

Over the course of the past few years, I have had several people ask me the same question: How did you come across this topic of research in special education and why is it of interest to you? This is the story.

It appeared to be one of those typical weary days in my life in which I was at the library engrossed and immersed totally and deeply in my doctoral studies. It was a day of thunderstorms. A gray overcast covered the skies of Pittsburgh. Of course, I was trying to track down the latest research in special education in preparation for my comprehensive exams. The doctoral program at the University of Pittsburgh is anything but easy and preparing for comprehensive exams certainly contributed to my feelings of anxiety and stress. The point of the preparation was to help me become an independent, analytical thinker and learner, but on that day I was not particularly interested in broadening my horizons. I was more interested in locating what I needed at the library and getting home to take a nap. Little did I know that my work at the library that afternoon would change my life, forever.

I was investigating some of the critical issues in special education such as transition, litigation, dyslexia, learning styles, mainstreaming, and the link between juvenile delinquency and learning disabilities. As I scrolled down the computer screen for the most recent published research articles, I spotted a research report about children with leukemia who, after treatment for their cancer, had acquired learning problems in reading, mathematics, memory, and concentration. I stopped cold in my tracks and started to use the computer keyboard as if I was a high-tech engineer in computer science. With some patience and persistence, I managed to retrieve the complete reference for the article. It was research that had been conducted at St. Jude's Hospital in Memphis, Tennessee, by two doctors, Raymond Mulhern and Judith Ochs. To find the article itself, I would have to trek up a very big hill to the medical library. By now it was pouring down rain outside, but I seemed unaware of the rain or the dreariness of the day as I forged on to my destination. My heart was pounding with anticipation and a surprising sense of enthusiasm. I was soaked to the bone from head to foot when I reached the library, and I quickly recruited a library assistant to find the correct journal. As we came across the article in a pediatric oncology journal, we breathed a sigh of relief.

I began to read the article about children who survived cancer against many odds, but after accomplishing this magnificent feat, they experienced educational, psychosocial, and physiological problems. The article was full of graphs and charts and statistical data that verified the children's deficits. In the reference section of this article, I saw other medical articles on this particular issue. I persuaded my library assistant to help me find as many articles as we could on the topic.

After I returned home to a warm bath and a cup of hot lemon tea, I called my adviser, Dr. Naomi Zigmond, to inquire if she had ever heard of this research. She said that she hadn't but as advisers should do, she encouraged and supported me to learn more about it. She felt, perhaps, it would be beneficial to include this research as a topic for my comprehensive exams.

After a very restless night, I called St. Jude's Hospital searching for one of the physicians who had written the article. I never thought I would have the opportunity to speak directly to Dr. Mulhern on my very first phone call to the hospital. But to my surprise, he accepted my call and he took a lot of time in sharing what he knew about children who survived acute lymphoblastic leukemia (ALL) and who often acquired learning difficulties. He offered to send me all the articles that he had written on the topic, along with a reference list to other researchers' publications. What a generous and kind man Dr. Mulhern was on that day.

When Dr. Mulhern's package of articles and reference list arrived, I went to work reading, researching, and learning everything I possibly could absorb about the medical aspects of ALL, the educational tests used to document treatment effects, and the results of research on survivors. I uncovered more than 50 articles reporting a reliable and valid link between the treatment of ALL and long-term learning problems.

When I defended my comprehensive exams, my committee was interested and enthusiastic about this new work. One member of my committee, Dr. Nettie Bartel from Temple University, had done similar research with children with leukemia in Philadelphia, and she encouraged me to explore the area further in my doctoral dissertation. However, I chose to do something very different from the research studies I had read; I decided to do a qualitative study instead of a quantitative one.

Qualitative research in education was only starting to catch interest. This form of research was usually found only in anthropology, sociology, and psychology. However, I was intensely interested in the individuals beyond whatever test results they demonstrated. Test results seemed so "sterile" to me. They could not reveal the "heart" and "soul" of a person's experience. I felt it was important to examine, retrospectively, the experiences, perceptions, and reflections of survivors of childhood ALL, and to describe, by giving voice to survivors' views, the related educational, psychosocial, and physiological sequelae of treatment and to the problems of school reintegration.

I made an initial contact with a physician, Dr. Vincent Albo, a pediatric oncologist at Children's Hospital of Pittsburgh, and asked for his help. He is a man of gentle demeanor who felt my work was greatly needed, and he supported my efforts in conducting this research. He understood the need to bridge the gap between pediatric medicine and education. He understood that medical teams were getting these children to survive medically but that it was the responsibility of educational personnel to accommodate their ongoing needs posttreatment. He helped me by giving me access, in a confidential manner, to individuals who might be interested in contributing to such a project. The result was not only a doctoral dissertation, a federally funded grant from the Office of Special Education Programs, and journal articles, but also this book.

This book contains stories of nine individuals who were diagnosed with ALL at age 5–7 years, received either dual systemic therapy (chemotherapy and irradiation) or only chemotherapy. One individual had experienced a bone marrow transplant as a form of treatment as well. These nine individuals were now post–high school adults who shared their experiences, perceptions, and reflections of the transition from illness to treatment, from hospital to home and school environments, in an open-ended interview. My focus in this work was not to survey individuals who survived leukemia but to "mine" their experiences. Storytelling is a research methodology that is growing in popularity in disciplines. Psychologists, doctors, sociologists, anthropologists, and historians "have become interested . . . in narrative structure, genre, and symbolic interpretation once considered literature's domain" (Randall, 1984, p. 1). Rita Charon, a physician and medical educator, contends that "medical work is centered on telling stories and on hearing stories . . . stories allow us to see inside our patients' lives with a clarity equal to any medical instruments" (qtd. in Mishler, 1986, p. 152). Narration is seen as a form of conversation that gives understanding to the human experience. It is through storytelling that we can achieve an understanding of a person's behavior in relationship to their experiences. I used an open-ended, semistructured interview to provide these individuals with the opportunity to tell their story and to probe deeply into various areas but most especially school-related experiences.

I think that the nine stories contained within the pages of this book are incredible. There is something unique and inspiring about them. Each is a journey into serious dialogue with a person who has survived a life-threatening disease at a young age. These young adults turned a devastating experience into a defining moment in their lives. Each story is a personal and intimate look at how every life is different despite the commonalties. We can recognize ourselves in someone else when that person is not afraid to risk and to share, honestly. The individuals who told me their stories were not afraid to risk or to share; and they did it to help others. They should be admired and commended for their humane contributions to this book and hopefully to every person who reads it.

How could anyone meet, listen to, and write these stories and not be changed for the better by the experience? I have become a better and more tolerant human being since becoming involved with this work. I found this work unexpectedly, and it has changed the course of my life unexpectedly in a moment of epiphany.

Part I

Surviving

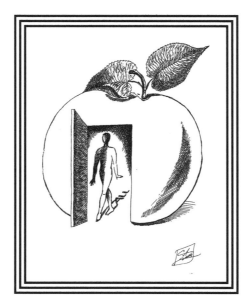

Life with and after Cancer: Walking with a Shadow

1

When Childhood
Leukemia Strikes

The childhood cancer experience has taught me many things.
However, if I had to choose one lesson learned along the way,
I'd have to say that I've learned that life is capricious; therefore,
we should make the most of every single day. Think about it: no
one knows what tomorrow will bring. It's not realistic for me to
say that I live each day as if it was my last. And yet, every
morning I remind myself to think this way.

—Honna Janes-Hodder

WHAT IS LEUKEMIA?

Blood is a very important substance that provides our bodies with oxygen,
food, hormones, and other chemicals. Blood removes toxins and waste
from cells and works with the lymph system to fight infection. Blood provides the cells necessary to repair injuries and to induce clotting. In a normal individual, healthy white blood cells are produced in the lymph
glands and bone marrow; they are the body's mechanism to defend
against infections and they trigger appropriate immune responses when
an infection invades the body.

Leukemia is a disease of the blood and bone marrow; diagnosis is usually
confirmed with a bone marrow aspiration (biopsy). In acute lymphoblastic
leukemia, the white blood cells (called "lymphocytes" or "lymphoblasts")

that are produced are abnormal or immature. They reproduce rapidly and flood the bloodstream. They interfere with the normal production of healthy white blood cells, platelets, and red blood cells. The extremely high numbers of abnormal white blood cells (often called "blast cells") flooding the bone marrow cause several serious problems. First, as normal white blood cells are being replaced by abnormal or immature leukemic cells, the body is more prone to infections. The leukemic cells lack the infection-fighting ability of normal white blood cells. Also, as red blood cells are being replaced by abnormal leukemic cells, the red blood cell count drops causing anemia; healthy red blood cells are essential for carrying oxygen to all parts of the body. The anemia that results from too few red blood cells causes weakness, fatigue, and a pale complexion. As abnormal leukemic cells continue to flood the system, the platelet count drops; platelets are tiny blood cells formed in the bone marrow that are essential for blood clotting. The result is excessive bleeding, bruising, and hemorrhaging. Finally, as abnormal white blood cells invade the blood-forming tissues, especially the bone marrow, they disrupt the normal production of blood cells. This causes swelling of the lymph nodes, spleen, liver, and kidneys. These symptoms of leukemia, including anemia (pale complexion), general muscle weakness, chronic fatigue, high fevers, bleeding (without clotting), bruising, recurrent infections, pain in the joints and bones, and swelling of the lymph nodes, spleen, and liver, are similar to those of many common ailments. So are other symptoms of leukemia: irritability, night sweats, fatigue, bone pain, and loss of appetite; headaches, poor work and school performance, weakness, seizures, vomiting, blurred vision, and difficulty maintaining balance. But in leukemia, these symptoms persist longer and eventually become quite severe.

Acute lymphoblastic (or lymphocytic) leukemia (ALL) can strike at any age, from infancy to old age, but about 80% of ALL patients are younger than age 15. Acute nonlymphoblastic leukemia (ANLL) is less common than ALL, affecting 1 out of every 100,000 children in the United States. ANLL attacks the white blood cells in the bone marrow that are not lymphoblasts, but it causes symptoms similar to ALL. The possibility of ANLL developing in a child increases throughout adolescence.

Another form of childhood leukemia is acute myeloid leukemia (AML) which is cancer of the granulocytes, another type of white blood cell. AML accounts for approximately 15% of all childhood leukemias.

There are also chronic forms of leukemia that progress more slowly than the acute forms. Chronic myelogenous leukemia is a disease that is usually associated with a specific chromosome called the "Philadelphia chromosome." If left untreated, chronic forms of leukemia can also be fatal.

It is estimated that 1 out of every 330 children in the United States will get cancer by the age of 19. In a school of 1,000 students, approximately 3 will be diagnosed with cancer (McDougal, 1997). Every school day, about 46 young people or two full classrooms of students, are diagnosed with cancer. In 2002, the statistics showed approximately 9,100 children from birth through age 14 were diagnosed with childhood cancer (American Cancer Society, 2002). Currently 12,500 adolescents are diagnosed with cancer annually (American Cancer Society, 2002; National Childhood Cancer Foundation, 2003).

Leukemia is only one of several childhood cancers, although it accounts for about 40% of all childhood cancers (Well-Connected, 2000, p. 1). Brain tumors have recently surpassed leukemia in children (Well-Connected, 2000). Nearly 4 in every 100,000 children between the ages of 2 and 10 are stricken with ALL, most of them between the ages of 3 and 7. In the United States alone, approximately 2,500 children are diagnosed with ALL each year, and the cancer incidence rate under age 15 appears to be increasing by 1% per year. Of course, the cure rate is increasing as well. Remission is declared when doctors cannot see any cancerous cells in the bone marrow when looking through a microscope, and across the United States nearly 75–80% of children with ALL go into remission. Currently, the 5-year survival rate for all childhood cancers is 77% (American Cancer Society, 2002). The cure rate is increasing by approximately 1.4% per year. It is estimated by the year 2010 that 1 in 250 young adults will be survivors of childhood cancer. Landers (2003) states, "Doctors now expect to cure three out of four children with cancer which translates to about one-quarter of a million such individuals in the United States now" (p. 2). Since the survival rates have increased, childhood cancer is seen as a life-threatening chronic illness rather than a terminal illness (Varni, Katz, Colegrave, & Dolgin, 1994). However, on a very serious note, even though survival rates have increased dramatically from 30% to approximately 80%, childhood cancer still stands as one of the leading causes of death in children aged one through adolescence (National Children's Cancer Foundation, 1997).

Childhood cancer has increased over the last 30 years. The number of ALL cases in children under age 15 rose by 27% between 1973 and 1990. Caucasian children are more likely to get ALL than African American children are, although socioeconomic factors do not appear to explain the differences. Boys have a slightly higher incidence of being diagnosed with ALL than girls do. However, girls tend to have more deleterious effects cognitively, psychosocially, and physiologically following long-term survival of childhood leukemia.

WHAT CAUSES LEUKEMIA?

> For those in whom cancer is already a hidden and invisible presence, efforts to find cures must of course continue. But for those not yet touched by the disease and certainly for the generations as yet unborn, prevention is the imperative need.
>
> —Rachel Carson, *Silent Spring*

Even though scientists and researchers know definitively some causes of childhood cancer, there are still many unanswered questions regarding why a child may develop cancer and, more specifically, leukemia. Studies have shown that childhood leukemia is not contagious and it is not usually inherited except through some genetic disorders.

There is some evidence that leukemia may result from a change in the structure of a gene that results in the abnormalities and uncontrolled multiplication of immature, abnormal white blood cells. According to research conducted at St. Jude's Children's Hospital (Steen & Mino, 2000), "Gene alterations have been observed in more than 90 percent of all human cancers, which strongly suggests that cancer results from a genetic change in cells" (p. 3). ALL has been associated with a number of genetic mutations. About 20% of adults and about 5% of children with ALL have a genetic abnormality called the Philadelphia chromosome. Children with this chromosome tend to acquire a more severe form of ALL. But up to 65% of leukemias contain some form of genetic rearrangements, called "translocations," in which some of the genetic material (genes) on a chromosome may be altered, or shuffled, between a pair of chromosomes. Why do these translocations or chromosomal aberrations occur? We can only speculate.

Several environmental factors may make a person more susceptible to leukemia, such as exposure to benzene (a flammable liquid obtained chiefly from coal tar for chemicals, dyes, and as a solvent), herbicides (a substance for killing plants, especially weeds), and pesticides (a chemical for killing pests such as insects or fungi). Recently, a study was conducted of three Irish counties in Ireland, which revealed that exposure to agricultural chemicals was associated with a high incidence of chronic leukemia and non-Hodgkin's disease, particularly in farmers who had not worn protective masks when spraying the pesticides (Well-Connected, 2000).

X-rays and other forms of radiation such as that released by atomic bombs during World War II on Hiroshima and Nagasaki, Japan, may also increase susceptibility to leukemia. On those Japanese islands, there was a 30-fold increase in the incidence of leukemia. Ionizing radiation, which includes x-rays and gamma rays, has so much energy that the rays can pass through the human body and disrupt chemical bonds. Increases in the incidence of leukemia have also been reported in Chernobyl in the Ukraine where a nuclear meltdown occurred at a nuclear power plant, and in Three Mile Island, Pennsylvania, the scene of another nuclear power plant mishap.

Viruses are suspected, because retroviruses or RNA tumor viruses have been linked to certain leukemias in animals. Some experts believe that some cases of childhood ALL may result from an abnormal response to infections. Clusters of ALL in children have been observed in different small geographical areas, and a recent Swedish study reported a higher prevalence in densely populated areas than in other parts of the country (Well-Connected, 2000). Curiously, children from affluent backgrounds, who do not attend day care, have a higher rate of leukemia. These children may not have had the exposure to viruses from being around groups of children that would lead them to develop stronger and more resistant immunity systems.

Family order, inherited genetic disorders, and being an identical twin with a twin who has ALL can play a factor in acquiring ALL. Some research has shown that a child born after another sibling is more likely to develop leukemia by the age of two or three than the firstborn or an only child. The fourth child in a family is at highest risk. (This is substantiated with the 9 stories in this book—5 out of the 9 respondents were the youngest out of 4 children.) However, even though siblings of a child with leukemia have a higher risk of acquiring the disease, there is a 1 in 500 chance, which is low incidence. But if one identical twin acquires leukemia, the other twin will have a 25% chance of also acquiring the disease within one year. Last, there is a 1 in 20 chance of a child inheriting ALL through mutations—defective genetic instructions passed down from parents to children. This can be evident in genetic disorders such as Down syndrome, Fanconi anemia, neurofibromatosis, Bloom syndrome, and Shwachman syndrome. For example, children with Down syndrome have a 20-fold greater risk of developing ALL than the general population (Well-Connected, 2000).

Influences at or surrounding birth have been associated with a higher probability of acquiring leukemia. One study found that infants whose mothers drank hard liquor during the second and third trimesters of pregnancy had more than a 40% increased risk of developing ALL; more than four drinks a month put the infants at greatest risk (Well-Connected, 2000). In the same study, fathers who smoked appeared to increase the risk for ALL in their children by 45% (Well-Connected, 2000). Another study reported that infants of mothers who were exposed to secondhand smoke during pregnancy showed more genetic abnormalities indicative of ALL than in babies who were not exposed (Well-Connected, 2000). According to Sandoval (2001), "Some oncologists believe that viral exposure while the child is still in the mother's uterus sets the stage for leukemia formation" (p. 2). Current research has uncovered "identical leukemia markers at diagnosis and from newborn screening samples" (Sandoval, 2001, p. 2). Investigation needs to continue in this interesting area.

Last, children who have been given chemotherapy and radiation for Hodgkin's disease are placed at a higher risk for acute leukemia within 2 to 13 years after treatment.

HOW IS LEUKEMIA TREATED?

> When I teach cancer pharmacology to second-[year] medical
> students, I always put a blowtorch on the table and say,
> "There's no cancer I can't kill. I'm not trying to be trivial, but I
> want to make the point that we don't treat cancer, we treat
> kids and we always worry about what we're doing."
>
> —Barton Kamen, MD, PhD, Professor of Pediatrics, Cancer
> Institute of New Jersey, New Brunswick

Once a diagnosis of leukemia is made, the standard treatment is intensive chemotherapy to stop the production of the abnormal white cells (or blast cells) and to restore the body's capacity to produce normal, healthy blood cells. This initial stage of treatment, the induction phase, can last from a few days to several weeks, as long as it takes to destroy many of the abnormal cells and obtain a stable remission. Patients remain in the hospital during this phase because they often need red blood cells or platelets transfusions along with the chemotherapy. Most induction programs include the drugs vincristine, prednisone, and L-asparaginase. For high-risk patients, daunomycin is usually administered. Other drugs may be included as well. Vincristine is generally given as an injection once a week; prednisone orally two or three times a day for 28 days; and L-asparaginase every two to four days, subcutaneously, for several doses. This combination of drugs is less toxic than other forms of chemotherapy. For example, there is little or no nausea. But there are other side effects. Vincristine can cause temporary hair loss, a tingling sensation in the arms and legs, muscle weakness, and constipation. Prednisone can cause an increase in appetite, weight gain, and a puffy appearance, and may affect blood sugar levels. L-asparaginase can cause pancreatitis, diabetes, and abnormal clotting or allergic reactions. But despite these side effects, 95% of children with ALL who receive three or more drugs during induction achieve a complete remission (Keene, 1999).

Once a stable remission is achieved, the induction phase continues, on an outpatient basis, with a treatment called the "central nervous system (CNS) prophylaxis." It is both a preventative treatment and a therapy designed to kill any ALL cells that may be hiding. Since the early 1970s, scientists have known that ALL cells were able to "hide" or find "sanctuary" in the brain, the spinal cord, and the male testes and, thus, escape the effects of the standard chemotherapy. CNS prophylaxis consists of combinations of the drugs methotrexate, cytosine arabinoside, cytarabine, and hydrocortisone injected directly into the spinal column (intrathecal chemotherapy), and radiation may be administered to the head, spinal cord, and, in boys, to the genital area. It was the discovery of the drug methotrexate 50 years ago that marked the beginning of survival in pediatric leukemic patients. With the addition of spinal injections and total body irradiation to the more standard chemotherapy treatment regime for childhood ALL, survival rates began to increase significantly. Unfortunately, the CNS prophylaxis treatment is also associated with many side effects such as stunted growth; poor enamel and root formation of teeth, gum disease, dry mouth due to salivary gland dysfunction; renal (kidney) complications; adriamycin-induced cardiac (heart) problems; endocrine problems (glands/hormones) in both boys and girls that result in precocious puberty or later infertility; motor disabilities; cisplatin-induced hearing loss; cataracts; and methotrexate-induced cognitive/learning difficulties (Thompson et al., 2001).

Oncologists are trying to reduce the neurocognitive deficits associated with dual therapy (chemotherapy and cranial irradiation) by only administering intrathecal methotrexate without cranial irradiation, or by reducing cranial irradiation from 2,400 cGx to 1,800 cGx in conjunction with intrathecal methotrexate. However, there is research evidence that between

40% and 70% of children treated with 1,800 cGx cranial radiation will still eventually acquire cognitive deficits. Any amount of radiation to the head area may cause lower brain processing speeds, greater drops in IQs, and the child's affect can change where the face appears expressionless (Candlelighter's Childhood Cancer Foundation, 2003). Currently, there is some research that has shown that only administering methotrexate or intrathecal methotrexate, due to its neurotoxicity alone, without cranial ir-radiation can also cause some more subtle, less severe, long-term learning and health problems.

The induction phase (chemotherapy and CNS prophylaxis) is followed by a second phase of treatment called "consolidation therapy or intensified phase." Now high doses of drugs that were used during the induction phase or a new and different combination of drugs are given orally, intra-venously, or intramuscularly. Currently, the drugs of choice are: methotrex-ate, cytoxan (also known as cyclophosphamide) or endoxan, cytosine arabinoside, 6-MP (6-mercaptopurine), dexamethasone (decadron), as-paraginase, and thioguanine. CNS prophylaxis can also be used during this second phase of treatment. The purpose of this second phase is to eradicate any leukemic cells that might have been left behind. Side effects and toxic-ity vary according to the dosage. However, reactions often include nausea, vomiting, mouth and throat sores, hair loss, and a temporary change in urine color to red or orange.

The final phase of treatment, the maintenance phase, consists of chemotherapy on a less intensive basis (once a week, once a month, then once every other month) for as few as two years and as many as five years. Typically, 6-MP is taken in the evening and methotrexate is taken weekly. Vincristine, prednisone, or dexamethasone may also be administered. Sometimes, methotrexate may be given intrathecally. It is not unusual for girls to receive treatment for two years and for boys to receive treatment for three or more years. The purpose of the maintenance therapy is to de-stroy the small number of residual ALL cells before they have a chance to multiply. Samples of blood, bone marrow, and cerebrospinal fluid are ex-amined periodically. Patients are monitored closely for any recurring dis-ease. If ALL recurs in the central nervous system or throughout the body, treatment consists of the CNS prophylaxis therapy plus treatment with the same or different combinations of drugs designed to induce a second, third, or even a fourth remission.

For some patients and their families, a clinical trial may be an option. A clinical trial is a research study in which human subjects participate to help scientists answer specific questions. A trial can test a promising new treatment, improve the results or reduce the toxicity of known treatments, or fine-tune existing treatments. Seventy-five percent of children with cancer are enrolled in clinical trials at some point in their cancer experience. The enormous improvements in treating childhood leukemia in the past few decades are the direct results of clinical trials. Every child enrolled in a clinical trial, while receiving the standard of care, is making a contribution to scientific research. Reference to resources in locating the newest treatments and clinical trials can be found in Appendix 5 under PDQ (Physician Data Query) and a cancer Internet Web site.

In addition to standard treatments of radiation and chemotherapy, advances in biomedical science and technology have also contributed to dramatic improvements in the long-term prognosis of children diagnosed with childhood cancer. One such biomedical technological advance is the bone marrow/stem cell transplant. In a bone marrow transplant, the patient has all of his or her stem cells removed from the bone marrow and the bloodstream. The patient then receives high doses of chemotherapy and sometimes radiation to destroy any remaining cancer cells. This process also destroys normal cells as well. After the patient undergoes these treatments, he or she receives an infusion of replacement stem cells, which may come from the patient, a relative, or an unrelated donor. Immediately after the transfusion, the stem cells do not function normally; it can take two to four weeks before normal bone marrow begins to develop. During this time, the patient must stay in protective isolation to avoid infection that he or she cannot fight. The patient is also at risk for serious complications or death due to the initial high-intensity therapy, from donor rejection or mismatch, or from graft-versus-host disease—a complication that occurs when transplanted cells attack healthy tissues.

Bone marrow transplants were started at a few hospital sites in the late 1960s. After decades of learning, it has been found that bone marrow transplants are not the be-all and end-all; they do not always produce a long-term cure. Instead, oncologists have discovered that some leukemic cells can actually survive the chemotherapy and radiation given preparatory to the bone marrow/stem cell transplant (just as some leukemic cells survive induction phase treatments by hibernating and then infiltrating the central nervous system or males' testicles). Unfortunately, these leukemic cells can actually infiltrate the new healthy graft-versus-host disease, transplanted bone marrow. Interestingly, a variation of the deadly graft-versus-host-disease, what researchers call "graft-versus-leukemia effect," might be the death knell for these persistent leukemic cells (Spice, 1997, p. C-2). It's a "high-wire act" that doctors and patients perform without a net—and, for now, without knowing just how wide or how long the tightrope might be (Spice, 1997, p. C-2).

When bone marrow transplants and total body irradiation are used together, certain side effects can be expected: thyroid dysfunction, growth delay, problems with sexual dysfunction and fertility, and cataract development. Other long-term side effects can include scoliosis, dental and facial problems, cardiac abnormalities, pulmonary abnormalities, liver damage, and urinary tract problems.

The preparation regimes for bone marrow/stem cell transplants have been know to be aggressive and harsh on a patient's body because of the toxic agents used to rid the body of any remaining disease.

*Bone marrow is spongy tissue found in the cavities of the body's bones where all blood cells are produced. A **bone marrow transplant** is when **stem cells are removed from the bone marrow for transplant.** Stem cells are considered the "parent cells." Every type of blood cell in the body begins its life as a stem cell. Stem cells divide and form new and different cells that make up the blood and immune system. These cells are found in both bone marrow and circulating blood. A **stem cell transplant** is when **stem cells are removed from the blood,** and returned after high-dose chemotherapy. (National Bone Marrow Transplant Link, 2001, pp. 20–21)*

Bone marrow/stem cell transplants have been used to "treat specific cancers in children such as leukemias, lymphoma, and neuroblastoma" (Children's Cancer Web, 2003, p. 1). Researchers are continuing to investigate using transplants for other types of cancer. Stem cells can be harvested from three known sources: bone marrow, peripheral blood (circulating blood of red cells that carry oxygen, white cells that fight infection, and platelets that are clotting agents), and the umbilical cord (rich in stem cells and obtained at birth). The following bone marrow/stem cell transplants have been the typical standard options for patients and families in curing cancer:

- **Allogeneic transplant:** Bone marrow or stem cells are donated by a closely matched family member, usually a brother or sister, or a closely matched unrelated donor. Genetics and ethnic background may have an effect on the likelihood of finding a donor.
- **Autologous transplant:** Patients donates their own bone marrow or stem cells prior to treatment for reinfusion later after high doses of chemotherapy or radiation.
- **Syngenic transplant:** Bone marrow or stem cells are donated by an identical twin.

There can be several side effects of having a bone marrow or stem cell transplant. Some of the side effects include: infection (caused by an immune system deficiency), hemmorrhage (caused by a lack of platelets), and organ damage (caused by chemotherapy or radiation). Graft (donor) versus host (patient) disease (GVHD) only occurs in allogeneic transplants and it can be from mild to life threatening. GVHD occurs when the body thinks the new stem cells are foreign and it starts attacking the tissues and organs.

Currently, there are some new types of transplants on the horizon, but they are specific to the age and the health condition of the patient. The following are fairly new types of transplants as described by the National Bone Marrow Transplant Link:

- **Non-myeloblative transplant (mini-transplant):** Blood stem cell transplant that uses lower doses of chemotherapy and radiation to prepare the patient for a transplant. Donor's cells and patient cells coexist in the body but work together to fight cancer cells. The procedure is less stressful on the immune system and gives hope to those who were ineligible for a transplant. Unfortunately, it is only for patients who are 50 years old and older.
- **Non-myeloblative allogeneic transplant:** Cells are from a donor, not patient. This procedure may reduce the size of solid tumors in patients with the following: renal cell carcinoma, metastatic melanoma, colon cancer, ovarian cancer, autoimmune diseases such as scleroderma and lupus, and myelodysplasic syndrome.
- **Tandem autologous transplants:** Timed autologous transplant to provide maximum tumor kill. Stem cells are collected prior to the first transplant to rescue the patient after two sessions of high doses of chemotherapy.
- **Second transplants:** Recommended if the disease occurs following transplant or if the donor's cells do not engraph. There is an increased risk to the patient because of the high doses of chemotherapy and radiation or from a prolonged period of immunity being compromised.
- **T-cell depletion:** Process where certain kinds of white cells called T-lymphocytes (which cause GVHD) are removed from the donor's stem cells to decrease incidence of GVHD and increase survival.
- **Donor lymphocyte infusion (DLI):** New strategy for managing relapse after BMT for patients who have CML, AML, and ALL. There is no chemotherapy or radiation prior to this therapy. DLI does pose

significant risk for GVHD and low white blood cell count that increases the susceptibility for infection and bleeding. (2001, p. 17–18)

Research shows that there are even more new treatments coming on the horizon that are being investigated in the area of DNA technology (gene testing). This research is showing great promise in determining what exactly triggers malignancies in the body's cells. (National Bone Marrow Link, 2001).

A relatively new drug called Gleevac was approved by the Food and Drug Administration in May 2001. Gleevac is to be used for chronic myeloid leukemia (CML), which can be a life-threatening blood disease. CML occurs when there is an overproduction of abnormal white blood cells in the body that live longer than normal cells. Gleevac turns off an enzyme that causes white blood cells to become cancerous and multiply. CML affects between 5,000 and 8,000 people each year. This drug can be used with adult or pediatric patients who have CML. It has worked with remarkable results to date.

SURVIVING CHILDHOOD LEUKEMIA

> . . . research indicates that individuals who have had
> cancer as children need to receive regular, life-long
> evaluation, and physicians need to be aware of the risks
> and potential of problems that childhood cancer survivors
> face. It is our hope that survivors who receive regular
> follow-up and support will experience fewer problems
> and disabilities related to their cancer treatment.
>
> —Dr. Charles Sklar, Medical Director of Long-Term Follow-
> Up Program, Memorial Sloan-Kettering Cancer Center

At one time, childhood cancer was the number one cause of death in children. From 1960 to 1970, the survival rate for children with leukemia was only 4%. By 1989, the survival rate had risen to 50%. By 1997, it was 79%. As recently as December 1997, Dr. Vincent C. Albo, pediatric oncologist at Children's Hospital in Pittsburgh, Pennsylvania, stated, "Never did I think that in my lifetime I'd be able to say to a parent: 'Your child will survive . . .' When I had to tell parents that their child had leukemia, the next sentence always was: 'He is going to die'" (personal communication). With prompt and aggressive treatments, most children with ALL are likely to survive at least five years, many living disease-free well into adulthood. Long-term survival for ANLL is 35% with chemotherapy alone, and increases to 50–70% when allogeneic (matched sibling donor) bone marrow transplant is conducted following initial remission. When long-term survival is achieved, entire lifetimes are saved. But surviving leukemia takes its toll—survivors' lives are changed forever by the disease.

Many adults who are treated for cancer and who are survivors of cancer resume their precancer lives and return to their workplace. Now that young children are finally surviving leukemia, they, too, are trying to resume a normal life and that includes returning to school. However, research results to date have indicated that the return to school and the ensuing few years are beset with problems (Sullivan, 1995; Sullivan, Fulmer, & Zigmond, 2000, 2001). Most young survivors report a strong need to return to a "normal life," to be treated normally, and to be just like their peers (Sullivan, 1995; Sullivan, Fulmer, & Zigmond, 2001). The majority of school-age children now treated for acute lymphoblastic leukemia return to school when they are released from the hospital after the induction phase of treatment. They are in school while they continue to have chemotherapy and, if prescribed to their protocol, radiation treatments on an outpatient basis for the next two to five years.

But returning to school is not easy. There are issues of school days missed and work to be made up. For some children, the induction phase of treatment may last several months, and for others, an entire school year may be lost. The child who survives the first stage of treatment returns to school lagging far behind his or her classmates academically.

Once back at school, there are still chemotherapy sessions, radiation treatments, spinal taps, and bone marrow biopsies to be endured on a regular basis. These painful procedures and anticipating them can certainly preoccupy a child's mind while classmates are paying attention to the teacher or the lesson. For example, if the hospital appointment were scheduled for Thursday afternoon, it would not be surprising if a child's concentration were very limited on Wednesday afternoon and Thursday morning, in anticipation of the hospital visit. It would also not be surprising if a good part of Friday is spent feeling the aftereffects of the procedures. Chemotherapy may cause fatigue, decreased energy, motor weakness, hearing impairment, and irritability (Armstrong & Horn, 1995). Paying attention in school can be very difficult under these stressful circumstances.

Next, there are inevitable psychosocial problems. Friends, or perhaps their parents, may be afraid because they worry that the disease is contagious. Or there is the child's embarrassment of losing his or her hair, of being too sick. A study conducted by Sullivan, Fulmer, and Zigmond (2000) supported past research that found children with cancer may experience further psychosocial issues in school. These issues included peer relationship problems, withdrawal from emotion, fear of trying new things, panic, stress, frustration and discouragement due to academic difficulties, and not feeling part of the group because of repeated absences.

School can actually be a dangerous place for the child survivor. Chemotherapy reduces the child's capacity to fight infection; common illnesses and infections become serious threats to the child's health. There are the constant dangers of catching colds or getting pneumonia. Exposure to chicken pox or measles can be lethal. Even scratched knees and bruises need to be given serious attention.

Finally, although cranial irradiation with spinal injections of chemotherapy is a critical component of the treatment for ALL, researchers have shown that this dual therapy can, itself, cause problems in the developing child. Without this dual therapy, patients run a greater risk of relapse that certainly threatens long-term survival; with this type of therapy, survivors run the risk of serious long-term effects including school learning problems. Brain irradiation has been proven to be an effective treatment but with this kind of therapy it brings with it a host of other issues such as learning problems, hormone deficiencies, and brain tumors. There is current research being conducted to learn if brain irradiation can be terminated effectively and safely as part of the treatment protocol of leukemia treatment. By eliminating this part of treatment, it would lessen the side effects for long-term survivors. Interestingly, it has been shown that methotrexate given intrathecally without irradiation to the brain can also cause long-term learning difficulties.

The statistics speak of more and more children surviving cancer, so it is imperative that the community who cares for these survivors are aware of their risks for late effects so that they have access to and can benefit from early intervention (Marina, 1997). Surviving childhood cancer long term can mean neuropsychological and cognitive deficits that are pronounced enough to impact a person's future academic performance, employability, access to insurance, and quality of life (Roman & Sperduto, 1995; Armstrong, Blumberg, & Toledano, 1999). McDougal (1997) states that these children are able to continue normal lives during and after treatment but as a community we need to provide support to them. Thus, research related to the effects of cancer and cancer treatment and how they affect the child's ability to carry on a normal life has become increasingly more important.

THE STORIES OF SURVIVORS

> She was the first person I had met who had survived it,
> and I cannot begin to tell you what difference that made.
> During my treatment, I just kept thinking about the woman
> who looked so healthy and vibrant and had lived a
> wonderful life, and this gave me hope.
>
> —Susan Fischer, cancer survivor,
> Memorial Sloan-Kettering Cancer Center
> "Patients Helping Patients Program"

> By walking with them through the clinic, to surgery, and then
> beyond to a "normal life," I have been able to help them see
> the light at the end of the tunnel. And they, in turn, have
> helped me. This experience has been so rewarding.
>
> —Bart Frazzitta, cancer survivor,
> Memorial Sloan-Kettering Cancer Center
> "Patients Helping Patients Program"

In numerous research studies published in medical and educational journals, scientists have documented the long-term effects of the dual therapeutic intervention of chemotherapy and radiation. The long-term effects relate to learning: problems in mathematical reasoning, reading problems, visual-spatial problems, memory problems, spelling problems, attention/concentration problems, distractibility, impulsivity, and problems in motor control (Bartel & Thurman, 1992; Sexson & Madan-Swain, 1993; Mulhern, 1994; Marina, 1997). When children survive the ravages of cancer and its conventional treatments, they can acquire a decline in mental functioning, IQ, and academic achievement (Thompson et al., 2001). Researchers have started to investigate the probability that academic performance may significantly be impacted by the neurological effects of the disease and treatment, a decline that can occur two to four years after the initial phase of treatment that closely resembles a nonverbal learning disability (Rubenstein, Varni, & Katz, 1990).

In almost all of the studies, large numbers of children diagnosed with ALL and treated with defined protocols of chemotherapy and radiation are given a variety of medical, psychological, and educational tests. Then the results are aggregated, subjected to statistical analyses, and reported to the scientific and medical communities. Researchers show that the extent of the physical, psychosocial, and cognitive deficits resulting from the treatments for ALL are related to the age of the child being treated (the younger the child, the more serious the deficits). Also, causing the extent of side effects can be the gender of the child (generally girls have more problems than boys), female cancer survivors tend to have 20% likelihood of more general health problems and 60% more likelihood of suffering from stress and anxiety long term (Marina, 1997). The higher the dose of chemotherapy or radiation given to a patient, the greater the risk for problems. Researchers document learning deficits, school-related difficulties, and social and emotional problems that all appear to affect a child's ability to reintegrate into the school environment after treatment. Some of the effects emerge immediately upon return to school; some are late in emerging, appearing several years after the child's treatments have ceased. Childhood cancer survivors typically have lower educational attainment.

But research results are cold and impersonal. They are numbers, statistics, and averages. They do not tell what it feels like to be sick, what it feels like to get well, what it feels like to return to school after this life-changing illness. They do not tell what the patients themselves perceive about their environments—hospital, home, and school—and about the changes in their lives, their recovery, and their return to a normal life.

That is the void this book attempts to fill. This book liberates nine young adults who are long-term survivors of childhood acute lymphoblastic leukemia by providing an arena to tell their stories. Although the individuals were diagnosed and treated for ALL 10 to 30 years ago, the stories within this book are timeless. Even though some chemotherapy agents and radiation doses have changed in treating ALL, what does not change is being a child with a family who experiences this life-altering trauma. Children are still continuing to be diagnosed and in greater numbers today. It truly does not matter whether it was 30 years ago or today because the pain, numbness, and fear of the unknown is still the same for the parent who hears that his or her child has cancer or the child who must go through the treatments. Whether a child had leukemia 10 to 20 years ago or today, the child as a survivor will go to school during treatments and after the treatments have ended. One of the changes in the past 30 years is that the 5-year survival rate is now approximately 80%. This is phenomenal compared to 4% in the early 1960s. However, even today, 15–20% of children diagnosed with ALL will not survive this insidious disease.

The chemotherapy drug methotrexate is still used today and can have long-term effects due to its toxicity on the nervous system. Although cranial irradiation is still considered a treatment option today depending on the child's medical status, it is used less frequently and when used the dosage is less than it was 10–20 years ago. However, with any cranial irradiation whether it is for ALL or brain tumors, it can still cause long-term neurological and cognitive difficulties for up to 10–15 years posttreatment. Lastly, today, there are antinausea and diarrhea medications to help prevent these side effects of chemotherapy or radiation either from occurring or reducing their impact during treatment. But nausea and diarrhea continue to be considered a side effect of treatment even though there are medications to help children not experience these side effects or to experience them in a lesser degree.

The nine stories were gathered through lengthy, semistructured interviews conducted over a period of several years. Also, the respondents' medical records at Children's Hospital of Pittsburgh were reviewed at great length and information from the records was integrated into the stories. Four of the stories (Frank, Elaine, Timothy, and Matthew) were collected as qualitative data for my doctoral dissertation (University of Pittsburgh) entitled *Educational Implications of Surviving Childhood Acute Lymphoblastic Leukemia and Its Treatment Regimes: Perspectives and Reflections of Long-Term Survivors.* Five of the nine stories (Patricia, Lynn, Ruth, Karen, and Joseph) were collected as qualitative data for one segment of a field-initiated federal grant. The grant was issued from the U.S. Department of Education, Office of Special Education Programs, Washington, DC, and awarded to me and my colleagues. It was received by the University of Pittsburgh and was entitled *Educational Implications of Surviving Childhood Acute Lymphoblastic Leukemia.* Both studies were approved with human subject clearances through the Human Rights Committees at Children's Hospital of Pittsburgh, Pennsylvania, and the University of Pittsburgh, Pennsylvania.

Through a pediatric oncologist, Dr. Vincent Albo, at Children's Hospital of Pittsburgh letters were sent to childhood acute lymphoblstic leukemia survivors who survived 10 or more years. To ensure the confidentiality rights of the patients, letters soliciting their participation in the studies were sent by the pediatric oncologist. If the individuals were interested in participating in the studies, they notified the oncologist who forwarded the information to me so that I could contact them. The criteria to participate in the studies was that each person had to have been diagnosed with childhood acute lymphoblastic leukemia between the ages of 5 and 7 and were given dual therapy (inthetracal chemotherapy with cranial irradiation) or only chemotherapy, particularly, methotrexate. Each of the survivors volunteered to share his or her experiences, perceptions, and reflections of the illness and the years since the illness in a semistructured, open-ended, tape-recorded interview.

However, it should be mentioned that there is always a margin of human error when working with quantitative as well as qualitative data. With qualitative data, the margin of human error in a study could well be the issue of "selective memory" when the subject is a human being talking about an experience that was very traumatic in his or her life. But what stood out during the interviews with these individuals, were their vivid memories of people, experiences, sights, and smells. Van Dongen-Melman, a researcher from Sophia's Children's Hospital/Erasman University, Rotterdam, The Netherlands, discovered that from the ages of 3½ to 4 years old, children have direct memories of all that has happened, especially the painful examinations, treatments, and the stays in the hospitals. Stuber et al. (1997) found that children who survived the childhood cancer experience have the psychological outcome of viewing cancer and its treatment as potentially traumatic events. Therefore, selective memory could impact the survivor's perceptions on their current reality predisposing survivors to adaptive and maladaptive outcomes. The individuals who told their stories seemed to have come out for the most part on the side of adapting positively, being well adjusted and leading productive lives. Some of the survivors, even though it had been several years later, shared that they had sought some counseling because of survival guilt or that they had struggled with commitment in relationships, which may be considered a maladaptive outcome.

A major difference today compared to 30 years ago is the fact that several hospitals have started grassroots programs related to survivorship. One such program is at Memorial Sloan-Kettering Cancer Center in New York City. They have instituted Long-Term Follow-Up Program that is specific to meeting the healthcare needs of childhood cancer survivors. This program was developed in 1990 due to the dramatic increases in children surviving cancer long term and issues associated with survial. The program provides survivors with medical treatment, screening, counseling, education, and prevention.

I needed to live, but I also needed to record what I lived.

—Anais Nin

The purpose of the two qualitative research studies I conducted was to examine, retrospectively, the experiences, perceptions, and reflections of survivors of childhood acute lymphoblastic leukemia, and to describe from their point of view the long-term physiological, psychosocial, and educational consequences of cancer survival.

The results from the studies substantiated findings from the quantitative literature. Overall, the nine individual stories contained in this book reflect positive experiences associated with school. But all of the survivors believed the experience of having cancer as a child and surviving into adulthood had rippling affects; it remains a part of their life forever. The two studies asked the individuals who survived their battle with cancer to recount it. Survivors shared their experiences, perceptions, and reflections of the transition from illness/treatment/hospital to the home and school environments.

According to Ledoux (1993), storytelling gives the individual a sense of power over what has happened to them. It provides the storyteller with the opportunity to go deeply into their conscious and subconscious to face life's deeper meaning. Fobair (1996), editor of the magazine *Surviving*, feels that reviewing one's life helps the individual gain a sense of inner control and the healing of psychic wounds.

These stories provide very personal perspectives and reflections on the long-term and delayed neurological and cognitive deficits, physiological problems, school-related difficulties, and psychosocial problems that often result from surviving childhood ALL. Survivors share their memories of the transition from health to illness to treatment to recovery. They recount their perceptions of the transition from hospital to home to school. They describe what it all feels like, and what more could and should be done to provide them with a higher quality support system as they move through their lives. These stories, for the first time, give voice to survivors' views of the educational, psychosocial, and physiological side effects of treatment and to the problems of school reintegration. It is hoped that through these interpretations, the frustrating consequences of disability can be reduced.

The nine individuals whose stories are told in this book were diagnosed with ALL between the ages of 5 and 7. All received treatment at Children's Hospital of Pittsburgh, and all but one received dual systemic therapy (chemotherapy and irradiation). One female survivor, Patricia, did not have cranial irradiation but was given chemotherapy. Interestingly, another female survivor, Ruth, had achieved full remission for 7 years following the dual treatment regime only to relapse and be diagnosed again with ALL. However, the second time of being treated for ALL, this individual only received chemotherapy without cranial irradiation.

The group consisted of five females and four males of whom eight were Caucasian and one was African American. At the time of the interviews, the young survivors were between the ages of 18 and 34 and had all graduated from high school. Three individuals (two women and one man) were starting college; two other women had attended and graduated from college. Only one individual (a male) had married and had two biological children; the other eight respondents were single with no children. Only two of the women had been diagnosed as having a learning disability, although several of the other respondents felt that they, too, had noticeable learning difficulties even though they were not formally evaluated for a disability. They attributed their difficulties to the childhood leukemia experience. Some of the participants experienced, in varying degrees, symptoms of posttraumatic stress disorder, an outcome common to about 20% of adult survivors of childhood cancer (Nir, 1995).

The stories contained within this book are more than chronicles of illness and hardship; they are celebrations of resilience and life. People thrive on "comeback" stories because it gives us all hope. *Hope* is the most powerful word in the English language. Each story is unique, yet there are similarities in the struggles and the triumphs. To the extent possible, each story is told in the words of the storyteller.

Following are summaries of the unabbreviated stories contained in this book. The names of the storytellers have been changed to protect their privacy.

Frank is 20 years old. He lives in a small town and works three seasonal jobs, each of them sports-related. Frank was diagnosed with ALL at the age of six, in second grade. He was out of school for nearly a year, and received chemotherapy and total body radiation. Paying for his treatments placed a great financial burden on his family, but they were very open about the cancer, and local fund-raisers were held to provide assistance. Frank served as the local Leukemia Society mascot for several years; he met many sports celebrities and was featured in local newspaper articles. He remembers his cancer experiences as very positive, and then and now he maintains a very upbeat attitude and a very positive outlook on life. Frank believes that surviving ALL opened doors for him and contributed to the success he feels today.

Patricia, at 34 years old, is one of the oldest living childhood leukemia survivors in the Northeast. She was diagnosed with ALL at age six, before full body radiation was a routine part of leukemia treatment. Her treatment consisted of massive doses of oral and intravenous chemotherapy. Patricia remembers being very lonely during her long stays in the hospital, but she doesn't remember anyone ever talking to her about what she had or what was going on. Patricia experienced severe reading difficulties and problems in concentration when she returned to school and throughout the remainder of her schooling, for which she never received any special services. It was not until Patricia was 17 that her parents disclosed to her that she had cancer. Disclosure remains a very painful and confusing issue to her. A recent diagnosis of, and successful surgery for, cervical cancer brought back to the surface her constant fear of the cancer returning. "It's always there behind you," she says, "lingering like a shadow."

Elaine is 25 years old. Her early experience with cancer is the reason she is, today, a pediatric nurse and an active volunteer in the Make-A-Wish Foundation. Elaine was diagnosed with ALL at age six. Her treatment program of chemotherapy and total body radiation was riddled with complications—collapsed lung, septic shock, pneumonia, numerous infections—which left her with several unintended side effects: crooked spine, weakened left arm, short attention span, and severe nonverbal learning difficulties related to problems in visual-spatial reasoning. Elaine remembers that she had a very special relationship with her teachers throughout school, although she missed half of first grade for her initial treatments, then all of fourth grade because of a chicken pox epidemic among her classmates. She was a very bright child, but was confused and frustrated when her low nonverbal IQ test scores kept her from being admitted into the school's "gifted program." Elaine developed a very close relationship with her family during her illness—she would not sleep anywhere but her parents' bedroom until age 10—but in her adult life, she continues to have difficulties in establishing and maintaining personal relationships. Nevertheless, she appreciates life so much because of her early cancer experience, and she works hard to give back.

Timothy is a handsome 26-year-old, with a wife and two children. He was diagnosed with ALL at the age of 5, though he was not told until age 15 that his illness had been cancer. His treatments lasted for five years, and he describes the experience as "terrifying"—being left alone at the hospital, the spinal taps, the bone marrow extractions, the needles. School was hard; he missed a lot of days and he experienced short-term memory problems and reading problems. Classmates nicknamed him "Popeye" because he wore a sailor's cap to school to cover his bald head. Timothy tries to put the cancer experience behind him but he cannot; it is always with him, it makes him cautious, it affects his relationships, it influences his perspective on life.

Matthew is 27 years old, the youngest of four siblings. He was diagnosed with ALL at age seven. At the time, he and his family lived near a nuclear power plant, and Matt was not the only child in the neighborhood diagnosed with leukemia. Matt thinks, however, that he is one of the few who survived. He attributes his survival to several sources: the horrible treatments of chemotherapy and radiation that he had to endure; the calm, steady, and secure environment that his parents created for him during and after the treatments; the teachers who were like guardian angels looking out for him when he returned to school; the attempts by everyone around him to not make a big deal of his illness and allow him to be like everyone else, "just a kid." But he struggles to this day with "survival guilt" and a search for what it was that made the difference.

Lynn is 18 years old, and is attending a small college in Western Pennsylvania, preparing to be a teacher. She was diagnosed with ALL at age six and was treated with chemotherapy and full body radiation. Lynn's parents were a constant presence and support for her during her treatments, but they never told her she had leukemia. When Lynn returned to school, she had serious difficulties in reading and math, and eventually was diagnosed as having a learning disability. Her difficulties in reading comprehension and concentration still plague her in college. Lynn's experiences associated with surviving leukemia were so traumatic that she has difficulty talking about them, discussing them, reflecting on them; Lynn brought her mother with her to the interview because she had never talked to an outsider about the leukemia experience before.

Ruth is 25 years old and currently works at a local retail store. She was diagnosed with ALL at age seven, at the end of first grade. Ruth had fairly traditional chemotherapy with cranial irradiation treatments over the course of three years. Her remission lasted for seven years when, almost to the month of her last treatment for leukemia, she relapsed in 1985. Ruth was now 14 years old, in the ninth grade, and again diagnosed with ALL. The same kind of chemotherapy treatment was administered but this time without the cranial irradiation treatments. Then she had an autologous bone marrow transplant that was riddled with complications including Legionnaire disease and facial shingles. Nevertheless, Ruth became a high school cheerleader, was crowned homecoming queen, and won the St. Francis Health Foundation's Courage to Come Back Award for her determination to beat the odds. She graduated from high school, attended college (where she was diagnosed with a learning disability), and graduated from college. Ruth acknowledges that the cancer experience was "psychologically and emotionally demanding," and yet she also views it as being a "growing experience." Her parents insisted that she "Keep your head up high and smile!" She hopes to give back one day to children who have cancer and she says, "Giving is what makes us truly happy."

Joseph at age 20 is the only African American among the storytellers. He graduated from high school and will be attending college to major in physical therapy. At the time of the interview, Joseph was working at a local pizza restaurant. He was diagnosed with ALL at the age of seven, in the second grade. On the day he was diagnosed, his mother walked out, leaving Joseph at the hospital alone. As a result, during the trauma of his illness and treatments, Joseph also had to contend with foster care, social services, and custody hearings. Joseph's treatments consisted of the various chemotherapy drugs and cranial irradiation. His complete treatment program lasted four years. Joseph reports no major learning difficulties but says that he often "zoned out" in school, thinking about other things, and he frequently got into fights with his classmates who made fun of his bald head. Joseph is philosophical about his childhood cancer experience, ". . . something happens to you for a reason . . . for some people the purpose is good . . . for some, it's not. I feel my purpose was good. It taught and prepared me for life."

Karen is 18 years old, working part time at a bakery waiting to begin college in the fall. She wants to study biology. She was diagnosed with ALL at the age of six, in the first grade.

Her treatment consisted of chemotherapy drugs but no radiation. She was only in the hospital for 11 days for the beginning of her treatments—she continued to be treated on an outpatient basis for the next two years. She viewed these frequent visits to the hospital as an acceptable "routine." Reflecting back to those days, Karen feels that she "missed out on things" and was "left out" a lot. Her school adjustment was complicated by a move to a new school in third grade. "It was a big change. Too many changes for me," she recalls. The most positive experience she remembers is Camp-Can-Do where she learned that "something good can come out of having cancer as a kid." Today, Karen is trying really hard to "balance her life . . . and plan her future."

We can truly understand the difficulties these children
face when we are able to read their experiences, as
told in their own words.

—Honna Janes-Hodder

These nine individuals were not afraid to risk opening old wounds to share their experiences in the hope of helping others. There is something unique and inspiring within each of their stories. There are also sobering issues that each survivor had to contend with such as relationships with siblings, parents, family members and friends; whether to disclose the illness or keep it a secret; whether to be retained in a grade after missing so much school or promoted to the next grade with classmates and friends; and whether to be treated as "special," thereby acknowledging the disease, its treatment, and the aftermath, or to be treated as "ordinary, normal, just like everyone else." Each child and his or her family dealt with these issues the best way they knew how at the time. In reading the stories, it is clear that there are no right or wrong ways to get through the experience of childhood acute lymphoblastic leukemia. But if there are lessons to be learned from the experiences of others, who better to offer insights, explanations, and recommendations than childhood cancer survivors themselves?

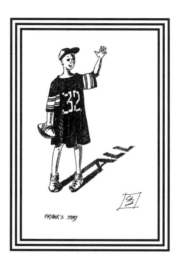

FRANK'S STORY

Sports Helped Frank During His Cancer Experience

2

What a Positive Experience!

Frank's Story

A consistent, positive attitude—making a stick into a
sceptre—allows us to turn an impossible situation
into a positive opportunity to find happiness.

—John Marks Templeton

Frank is a Caucasian male, currently 20 years old. He is the youngest in a
family of four siblings; he has three older sisters. Frank is average height, and
stocky. He gives the impression of being in good physical/athletic shape. His
brown hair is cut short. Frank lives in a small town north of Pittsburgh and
works three different seasonal jobs. He is an intern scout for the Pittsburgh
Steelers; he works at Dick's Sports and Clothing Store; and he helps in the
summer with the University of Pittsburgh's football program. Frank's jobs
keep him very busy, but he was pleased to have been asked to tell his story
and he made time for the interview. "If I can do something that would make
a difference in someone's life, then it's worth it." During the interview, Frank
was relaxed and calm, direct and open, with a sense of humor.

ONSET OF THE DISEASE AND TREATMENT

At the age of 6, in the fall of 1981, Frank was experiencing soreness in
his muscles and bones. Usually, when this had happened in the past, the

soreness was always associated with playing football and it would last only 2 or 3 days. This time, however, the soreness was chronic and incessant; it lasted nearly six weeks before his parents finally took him to see the pediatrician. "I was complaining."

Frank had just started second grade. The pediatrician diagnosed him as having a virus, and prescribed antibiotics as the course of treatment. After 2 weeks without any improvement, Frank's father took him to Children's Hospital of Pittsburgh. The medical record indicates that Frank was tested and that the doctors described his condition as progressive malaise and weakness. He had a temperature of 102°F with pronounced intermittent left shoulder, left leg, and right leg pain; he was also anemic. He had lost seven pounds in 2–3 weeks and was having night sweats and chills. Frank was discharged but within a very short time the hospital called his parents to bring him back immediately; they had found something.

Frank returned to Children's Hospital on November 5, 1981, and was diagnosed with childhood acute lymphoblastic leukemia. The spinal tap and bone marrow results (91% malignant cells) were characteristic of ALL. Frank remained in the hospital for the next 8 days. The first phase of his treatment (induction) began on November 6 and consisted of daily treatments of prednisone, vincristine, L-asparaginase, and intrathecal methotrexate. On November 10, Frank was also admitted into a research study for the drug bactrim. He was discharged on November 13 and continued daily outpatient treatments and an oral form of bactrim until November 27.

The second phase of treatment (intensified) began on November 27 and continued through December 18, 1981. Treatment included all the drugs from the induction phase plus 6-MP. In addition, Frank received radiation to the brain from December 9 through December 22; he had 10 treatments at 1,800 cGy. According to the medical record, the radiotherapy was given to him to prevent central nervous system relapse and Frank tolerated the treatments fairly well.

Frank's third phase of treatment (maintenance) began on December 28 and lasted for 2 years (to December 16, 1983). The maintenance phase chemotherapy included prednisone, 6-MP, vincrinstine, cyclophosphamide (cytoxan), methotrexate, and intrathecal methotrexate. At the 2-year evaluation, a testicular biopsy indicated that no tumors were present. Frank's total treatment regime lasted 3 years.

Frank's major medical complaint from the start of treatment to the present has been severe headaches: "I get bad headaches a lot but I suppose it's the effects of the drugs." A CT scan of the head, administered on December 1, 1994, after 15 years of severe head pain, revealed a slight prominence of the sulci and in the white matter of the left frontal lobe. The radiologist believed that it was probably caused by the previous chemotherapy and radiation, but there were no tumors. Frank has had no anticancer therapy on any follow-up visits since December 16, 1983.

FRANK'S REACTIONS TO DIAGNOSIS AND TREATMENT

During his first 6 days of treatment at the hospital, a female physician was in charge of his care. Frank did not like this doctor; his tone of voice changed when talking about her.

I hated the lady who was taking care of me. She was terrible. She didn't do anything right. Everytime she was trying to take blood, she couldn't. She wouldn't hit the vein. Every time she did a spinal tap, she wouldn't do it right. I kept saying I wanted to get rid of her. It had nothing to do with sex . . . a feminist thing or anything . . . the truth is the truth. It was a matter of care and treatment.

Frank blamed his mother for not doing anything about this terrible doctor.

That first doctor . . . I hated her and that made me hate my mom. Because I kept telling her to get rid of her. And she wouldn't do it. So I was mad at my mom for not taking control and doing something. It took that doctor a half an hour to just do the Novocain. And my mom was coming in, and I'm like get away from me. I didn't want her around me because I expected when I said something she should do it for me. It was hurting me.

By the sixth day of in-hospital treatment, a new, male doctor was assigned to Frank's care, and then

. . . as soon as the doctor was changed, everything was fine. . . . [H]e came in and took right over whatever she was doing at the time. He came in and said I'll do it. And he did it right away. Just like that. Just like he had his eyes closed. You could tell how much better he was at doing those procedures. You saw a great change in me then.

His parents and the doctors, as a team, told Frank about his condition and about the treatment it involved during his initial days of diagnosis and treatment. They told him "it was pretty serious." Frank "kinda made things light. I mean if you talked to any of the nurses that were there with me . . . they loved me . . . because I was funny. I made things fun. I wasn't a downer all the time." His parents didn't give him a choice about whether to have the treatments. He thinks that they knew what kind of person he was and they just went through with the treatments automatically, without hesitation or apprehension. "They knew how I was. They knew I would fight. They didn't seem too worried. They were only upset with my pediatrician that he didn't check very thoroughly. That's who they were upset with."

Frank didn't really appreciate the seriousness of his disease until one of his friends at Children's Hospital died.

My first day there [at Children's], he walked in. We weren't allowed to eat salt but this kid ate more salt things . . . he had Ritz crackers . . . the most salt thing in the world. So, he was eating them and we were watching TV. I told him, "Isn't this terrible . . . the leukemia?" He said "Yea." So, we talked and would go to the rec room down the hall. I didn't have any friends there. But it was cool because we used to play Connect Four. We were supposed to be in our rooms but we'd sneak down there. I think he left the same day I did but he had to go back. He had a bone marrow transplant but he had a reaction to it . . . some bacteria disease . . . it reacted to his body. It didn't work good. I was almost [in remission] and he was going down. I was supposed to go to his birthday party and my parents had to warn me he would be wearing an oxygen mask and they were unsure how comfortable I would be with that. Anyway, something else had come up and I couldn't go anyway. So, then a couple weeks later, I went to the doctors, and I saw his parents there. I'm like, "Hey, where's Sammy? I mean how is he doing?" They weren't saying anything. Then I got home and my Mom said he had died. It was kinda weird. See all this time I was getting better. I was like invincible, that nothing was wrong with me. People would pinch me with needles but I was made of steel. And then, one of my friends died. It brought me back to reality that this could happen to me. I knew then what I had was serious.

Once the initial phase of treatment was over, Frank would return to Children's Hospital every Thursday for cytoxan. To Frank, it was "a poison . . . it made me throw up really bad but by Friday I could eat again." Frank also remembers returning to Children's Hospital every 2 weeks for a spinal tap and a bone marrow biopsy.

I would go in every other Wednesday. I would get a spinal tap but the bone marrow was the worst. I didn't care about the spinal taps. I didn't care about anything else. It wasn't just that the bone marrow hurt but it was that you could hear it . . . the needle going into the bone . . . you could hear it crunching. They would just put Novocain in . . . you felt the pressure on the nerves, like at the bottom of your feet.

In addition to these hospital-based procedures, Frank's mother gave him "shots in his legs" at home, "but the needles didn't scare me." And he had to take as many as eight pills, including the cytoxan, every day.

Sometime during that period of time, Frank's sister came down with chicken pox. The chicken pox virus can be life threatening for chemotherapy patients who have a suppressed immunity system. So, Frank had to go to the hospital and "they gave chicken pox to me and I had hives in a matter of seconds so I would never get it."

TREATMENT SIDE EFFECTS

Frank experienced some mild side effects from the treatment regimes, particularly hair loss. But the hair loss was "no big deal," except when Frank went to church. "I am Catholic and the only time I felt uncomfortable was when I made my first Holy Communion. My hair was starting to come in . . . like peach fuzz. I wasn't allowed to wear my baseball hat in church."

Frank experienced some swelling because of the prednisone but as soon as he was off it the swelling disappeared. He experienced transient skin irritation, but overall, he tolerated the treatment regimes very well. And he was spared from two frequent side effects of treatment: sterility and stunted growth.

While Frank was hospitalized and during his subsequent trips to the hospital, Frank "became a star." Well-known people in sports and television visited him. Foge Fazio had become the football coach at the University of Pittsburgh and he took to Frank. Frank met members of the University of Pittsburgh's football team. It was "mandatory when you sign a contract to play for Pitt and if you're a big-time star or if you are acknowledged as one, then you have to go to Children's." Frank became the mascot for the team and for the Leukemia Society of Pittsburgh. He spoke at celebrity luncheons.

I was in the newspaper and everything. There was an article about me entitled "Gray Skies Can't Ruin Franky's Heroes." I received a TV from the tournament. I kept the clippings of when I was a mascot and I still have the book. Jim O'Brian was the sports information director [at the University of Pittsburgh] and I was put in the 1985 yearbook. That was when I was in third grade.

Players from the Pittsburgh Steelers, like Jack Ham, and players from the Pitt football team, like Dan Marino, visited with him regularly when he was hospitalized. "They gave out their practice jerseys. It helped me. It showed that the players didn't just care about themselves."

Frank was also visited by Fred Rogers from *Mr. Rogers' Neighborhood*, a television program that originates from Pittsburgh. Mr. Rogers did a Christmas special from Children's Hospital on CBS and Frank appeared on that show and was interviewed by Mr. Rogers. Frank believes he was chosen because

I was always positive and I have a good personality. Everybody liked my personality. They always said that I made people happy. That's why I became the mascot for the Leukemia Society and I was able to meet all these people.

IMPACT ON THE FAMILY

Frank's parents visited and stayed with Frank frequently. Frank's paternal grandfather, came often, too.

. . . he wasn't around too much when my father was younger. He admits he wasn't a good father, but he's been a great grandfather. We are buddies. It was my parents and him who came and took me places. No one else did.

Frank's mother worked as an aide at Mayview State Hospital, but took time off from work for a while during the initial stages of Frank's illness. His father had asked his boss to lay him off for a period of time, too. Frank's father is a title researcher and today has his own company. He is also a singer and, according to Frank, "one of the best in Pittsburgh."

Frank's "parents weren't too financially burdened" by the costs of treatment. There were donations made for Frank through the football programs. Also, one of his father's friends owned a bar and they had a fund-raiser there for Frank. Through various avenues, his parents were able to manage the extra costs.

Frank felt that through the entire ordeal his parents weren't too overly protective of him. Even though he was stricken with a serious illness, he had a minimum of restrictions. He stopped playing football for about a year, and he was not permitted to eat salt because of the prednisone that causes swelling in the body. He was not permitted to return to school for nearly a year.

When he returned home from the hospital, one of Frank's best friends in second grade was very distraught over Frank's illness and reached out for help to Frank's own mother. The friend

. . . sat down and talked to my mom. He only told me that when we got older. I think it [was] good [that] my mother [talked to my] friends. A mom can say, "Don't be afraid to come over and see him. This is what happened and it's not catchy."

Frank's three older sisters treated him "like normal." He was closest to the second oldest sister; she helped him a lot with school. "The first oldest and the third were too motherlike." Now he feels he is close to all three sisters.

His mother is Catholic and took him to church during his childhood. Today, Frank considers himself Catholic but not a practicing one. Frank has six nieces and nephews and he is godfather to three of them.

I take that pretty serious . . . being a godfather . . . that's supposed to be a holy thing. The thing is I'd go to church today but I feel bad I haven't. . . . I haven't told my sins . . . not since second grade . . . so it's something I'd like to do. I don't feel comfortable going . . . but I pray every night before I go to bed . . . sometimes when I eat. I believe but what got me off was I remember I wasn't in Catholic school and so I had to attend Saturday classes . . . CCD. Football was on Saturday and I could never go. I just made my confirmation at 18 years old.

Frank's family believes in God, but they just don't go to church. They aren't avid believers or very strict about it.

We don't eat meat on Good Friday and we go to church on Christmas . . . that's about it. I had to go to church when I was going to be a godfather. I don't think being Catholic had any part [in my remission; God] might just like me.

THE SCHOOL EXPERIENCE

Frank was diagnosed in November of his second-grade year of school. He didn't receive any tutoring or help with school while he was hospitalized. Once he came home, his second-grade teacher, Mrs. Morgan, came to the house three times a week, between December 1981 and April or May 1982. "She was my actual second grade teacher. She didn't live too close but I guess close enough." The school had not ordered tutoring for Frank. The teacher "didn't have to do it" but she did it anyway.

We would go over spelling and spelling tests. We'd read a book. We'd do a little bit of English, social studies, and science. But just a little at a time. I really hadn't lost much . . . just a lot of my own experiences being in second grade.

Frank enjoyed the tutoring experience. "I would get kinda bored being home and she was like my connection to the world outside."

This second-grade teacher also kept Frank in touch with his classmates. "She had the class make me cards and at Christmas they made and gave me a dollar tree. It was pretty cool."

Before the end of the school year, Frank's doctor told him it was time to go back to school. The nurses started to kid him about it, but no one really prepared him in any way to return. He just ". . . pumped myself up. I just sat there and talked to myself to get the adrenaline going. Maybe it was just my personality. I know I was excited to go back."

Two or 3 weeks before returning to school, the sister to whom he felt closest at the time, decided to make a cassette tape on which Frank could speak to the entire class. Frank recalls, "I said how I appreciated Mrs. Morgan coming to my house. I appreciate everything the class had done for me. And I said I'll see you guys in a couple weeks." His sister took it to school for him.

The reintegration was uneventful.

The kids were excited for me to come back . . . except the one girl who said something to me. Her name was Rose and that was ignorant. The only thing I wanted to make sure of was that they treated me like they did when I was in first grade. There was nothing different about me. I didn't need any help. I didn't have any anxieties about going back to school.

Frank didn't have any hair when he returned to school, but he wore a hat. "I wasn't anxious at all about somebody laughing at my hat. I was like if someone laughs, you know they are ignorant." He didn't have any trouble reestablishing friendships. "I was friends with everybody, or they were just afraid of me because I was the class bully. Most of my close friends were in first grade with me." Frank's parents were around at school, too, to make sure no one treated him differently. "If I got bad, I was disciplined. I was not paddled but if I got out of line, she [the teacher] would put you back in."

Mrs. Morgan did talk to Frank's parents about his condition and progress, but she never spoke to any of his doctors. In subsequent school years, Frank's teachers and his principal always asked him how he was doing; Frank felt they were just a little protective of him. It was a small elementary school so Frank knew everyone. Frank's mom had made sure that when he returned to school the staff knew about her son. Still, he did not receive any support help (including none from a school nurse or school psychologist) upon returning to school. He was placed directly back into second grade and despite having missed most of the school year, he was not retained.

Frank's parents appeared to value education even while Frank was ill. They would work with him at home between his teacher's visits. They would read with him or help him with an assignment. Frank's parents were

. . . concerned with my education even through the middle of this. They were still concerned. If I had a question, they would help me. My dad was good in reading and my mother was good in math. Also, my middle sister was smart. She always got the good grades out of all my sisters.

AREAS OF SCHOOL DIFFICULTIES

Initially, the reintegration into school went well, but Frank was never a very enthusiastic or successful student and "later down the road, school was putrid." He had the most difficulty in comprehension. "If I read a story, I wouldn't be able to concentrate." As far as the other subject areas, Frank "was never good in math or cursive writing" but long-term and short-term memory did not seem to be particularly affected.

Occasionally, Frank used his illness to get out of class.

I could have used it a lot more if I wanted to. I could have milked it more. In fifth grade, I know I milked it. Something happened to our teacher and she knew me well and then we got a different teacher. If I had to go to the bathroom, I would just walk out and not ask her. You know because I could say I had a problem. I did miss as much school as I could get away with.

But Frank never used his illness to stay home because his parents wouldn't permit it. So, if he wanted an excuse to stay home from school, he would simply miss the bus.

By fourth grade, Frank "just didn't want to be there."

I probably started cutting school at least twice a week. By high school, they have a truant officer . . . then I'd either go in the morning and leave or I'd come late for just the afternoon. I'd have them call my sister to ask if I could leave school and she would say yes. I would always miss every couple of Fridays [while in elementary school] because that was my checkup days at Children's."

After high school, Frank attended Community College of Allegheny County, majoring in psychology. However, Frank never completed the necessary course load for graduation. His current plan is to begin classes in the spring term at the University of Pittsburgh after he has completed his work related to the fall football season schedule. Again, he will major in psychology. "I chose psychology because of the way I am. It amazes me how a person can hear one thing and interpret it to mean something different. I always thought that was interesting."

SURVIVING

Frank believes that laughter is important to making yourself better. He says "to laugh about things, and make other people laugh . . . and have faith. The doctors know what they are doing or else they wouldn't be doctors."

Frank still goes to his same group of doctors for annual checkups. He says his doctor uses him as an example for other children being diagnosed with leukemia.

I'm kind of like a specimen. I was in the hospital for only 10 days and then I was in remission within a year. That might be a world record for leukemia. Now, when I am at the office, the doctor has me talk to the kids. I talked to one kid who was really scared . . . he was young . . . and I just sat there and talked to him . . . told him how to cope with it all . . . and that he can do it the way I did.

Frank recognizes that the leukemia experience was not always bad. "I am not a miserable person because of what happened to me." It "opened up doors" for him. "It was the beginning of a chain of events for me up to today. That's how I even got my job."

Having leukemia played a significant part in Frank's life. It helped him see that positive things can come from very terrible times. And now that he has learned that, he knows what he must do. "I don't mean to get back to religion, but I think God helped me and now it is my civic duty to help others."

3

Why Am I Here?

Patricia's Story

Numbers, science, and medicine all fail to answer
a deceptively simple question, "Why me?"

—Tom O'Connor

Patricia is 34 years old, the youngest of three sisters. She is of average height and has a chunky build. She wears no makeup; she likes the natural look. Her hair is brown and thin, and falls just to the top of her shoulders. She smokes a pack of cigarettes a day. "They [the doctors] tell me, you know, I have to quit. I've quit a couple of times. I am quadrupling my chances of getting cancer again. And even though I know this, I continue to do it. Go figure."

Patricia lives near Latrobe, Pennsylvania. She has worked various jobs, none of them requiring very much skill. Currently, she is a bindery worker in a check printing company. Patricia has worked there for 5½ years and she likes her job. "I'm good at it," she says.

Patricia is one of the longest living survivors of childhood leukemia from Children's Hospital of Pittsburgh. Her comments were astoundingly honest, open, and straightforward.

ONSET OF THE DISEASE AND TREATMENT

Patricia was diagnosed at the age of 6, while she was in the middle of second grade. It was 1966.

I had a fever of 104. It wouldn't go down. [My parents] must have called the hospital or the doctor. They [were] told [to] put me in a tub of ice. Well, they put me in the bathtub with all the ice in it but [the fever] still wouldn't go down. . . . So that's when they took me into the hospital and they kept me. They broke the fever. They ran some tests. They figured out I had leukemia.

The medical team started Patricia on a treatment regime immediately. She had intensive chemotherapy that consisted of prednisone and 6-MP, but no radiation. In 1966, dual therapy using chemotherapy and radiation had not yet been authorized as a standard treatment for ALL. At that time, survival rates for ALL were a mere 4 percent. "I took pills and some intravenous chemotherapy" for approximately 3 weeks, though she stayed in the hospital for just over 2 months. "The first phase of treatment was from February 21 to March 2, 1966. I went home from the hospital on the 30th of April. That was the last time I was in the hospital [for leukemia]." Maintenance therapy was in pill form and lasted for 5 years. Then, Patricia was on a long-term maintenance program that consisted of one mild chemotherapy pill every day from age 11 to age 17.

Once she was home, and back at school, Patricia came down with the measles, and was quarantined at home for several weeks. After that, her recovery was quite uneventful.

PATRICIA'S REACTIONS TO DIAGNOSIS AND TREATMENT

Patricia did not know that she had cancer at the time of its onset, diagnosis, and treatment. Her parents did not tell her of the leukemia until she was 17.

All those years, from age 6 to age 17, my parents didn't tell me the true reason I was sick. I just found out when I was 17 that I had leukemia and I was in remission.

The revelation made her resentful, because it made her feel that she, not just her parents, had been made to lie all those years.

I should have known. I mean, I lied like my whole school years. [When someone asked me], "Why was you sick?" I said, "I had pneumonia and I had measles at the same time." I mean, I didn't know the true reason.

Patricia remembers that she was very sick during those 3 months at the hospital. She remembers people being there, and lots of crying. "[The priest] gave me my death rights. I was to have only 3 weeks to live and that would be it. Well, everyone was like . . . devastated."

But the most pervasive memory of her hospital stay was of loneliness.

I was just so lonely. I mean, I remember lying there. My mom and dad had two other children. They couldn't be with me constantly . . . 24 hours a day. You know? [My sisters] were in school. I was at the hospital a lot by myself.

To keep her company, her grandparents gave her a small stuffed animal, a stuffed dog.

Well, that animal became my friend. I said everything to it. And, I held it, and cried on it. I slept with it. When they [my parents] would come, I'd be real happy. But then they'd be leaving, and I'd be bawling my eyes out again . . . my stuffed dog and me.

Patricia has never forgotten the procedures performed during her stay at the hospital.

Oh . . . them bone marrows. Oh . . . Oh . . . Oh . . . they were every month. They'd stick the needle in your hip and draw out the fluid. Then, . . . they put a needle in your back and draw out fluid . . . a spinal tap. We used to have to drive to Children's Hospital every month from [where we lived]. I'd cry cause I knew what was coming.

Nor has she forgotten the doctor who treated her.

My doctor, I must say, I loved him. He was great. He was really kind. He told me he wouldn't lie to me. They would prick my finger. They had to count the cells of everything once a month. He told me it would hurt, but he had to do it. He always told me what he was going to do. He apologized that he had to do it, but he had to make me better. He'd do it and it wouldn't take very long. As soon as it was over, I know he gave me treats after every procedure. Then I'd be on my way.

She also remembered one very unpleasant episode while in the hospital.

I remember this nurse coming in and she said, "You have to eat this Jell-O." And . . . I don't want to eat my Jell-O, you know. I didn't want anything. And she's [calling me] "bratty kid." . . . Well, I'm not eating it. So, she threw me in my bed, and that needle in my arm . . . came out. . . . My mom and dad came down that night. And I said that a nurse threw me in bed and ripped the IV out of my arm. It was bleeding where she knocked it. I never seen that nurse again the whole time I was in the hospital . . . whether they fired her . . . or just moved her . . . I don't know. I don't ever remember seeing her again.

TREATMENT SIDE EFFECTS

Patricia experienced all the usual side effects commonly associated with receiving any form of chemotherapy or steroids (prednisone) in the treatment protocol for cancer.

When I was in the hospital, having intravenous therapy, I remember I was a real skinny from throwing up. I was really skinny kid. But . . . like I have these pictures that [show] my face was all blowed up. I was a really small kid, but my face was real puffy from the drugs. It was funny looking.

Migraine headaches were a problem. "I do remember that I had a lot of them when I was little. It's from the drugs. That's what the doctors told me." Migraine headaches seem to be one of the long-term medical side effects of the chemotherapy regime.

And to this day, I still get them. This is kind [of] gross, but . . . the thing is to get rid of them I either have to throw up and/or go to bed . . . if you go to sleep and then you wake up, it will be gone. [The headaches] last about a day. I've noticed I had more when I was little. Now it is every 6 months or so. Then I'll get a major headache. I always have to have my warm ginger ale, too. It makes me throw up, then I feel better.

Patricia also complains about her susceptibility to colds and bronchitis, which she also attributes to the long-term side effects of chemotherapy.

I feel like I have a low resistance from being so sick when I was young. Those drugs they have you on can play havoc with your immunity system. If anybody is sick . . . I am definitely sure to get it. You know whether it be a cold, flu, or whatever I get it automatically.

Like most children who are treated for cancer, Patricia lost her hair during chemotherapy, but she said that it was no big deal.

I lost my hair when I was little going through the treatments. I don't recall ever wearing any hat, scarf, or wig. I don't remember anyone saying anything to me about having no hair either. It was just an acceptable fact of life at the time. There isn't anything you can do about it. Everyone just lives with it.

When her hair grew back, it seemed to have changed its texture. "I have thin hair today, but the hair on my legs grows very quickly and I have to shave all the time. My teeth and nails are pretty strong, though."

Patricia goes for annual medical checkups and is very vigilant about her health.

I try to make sure I get my blood work done every year, . . . because not only do I check it for leukemia, . . . but sugar [diabetes] runs in my family. So, I try to have both of them tests taken so that I know that everything is all right. I changed doctors and I had all my records sent to this one but he didn't meet up to my expectations. So . . . I changed to another doctor just a few years ago and I like him a whole lot. If I go there for any reason, he runs the test on me.

When she was 30, Patricia was diagnosed with cervical cancer. Laser surgery was performed and "they got it in time." Now, Patricia considers herself cured, "but every six months I go to my gynecologist to see if it has returned." Having experienced two kinds of cancer, Patricia worries about being sterile.

I always wanted to have children . . . but who knows? After having two kinds of cancer, I think there is a greater chance that I can't [have children] and that does bother me. I think when the option of your own personal choice is taken away, it makes it harder.

Yet, she hasn't undergone any fertility testing. "Why get tested until I am married and ready to make that decision or choice? It's senseless to worry about it until the time comes. Why waste the energy?"

IMPACT ON THE FAMILY

At the time of her illness, Patricia's father was a steelworker. Her mother may have worked at one time but Patricia remembers her being mostly at home. Her father was the strong one, not very emotional, trying to be "tough." Her mother was just the opposite: openly sad, and she would cry while visiting Patricia at the hospital. "My mom always looked like she was in agony. My dad was always kind of . . . tough, you know? My mom would cry but then my dad would take her away whenever she'd start [crying]."

Patricia doesn't remember her mother staying at the hospital overnight or on weekends. In her memories, her parents came to visit and then left. Of course, she realizes now that she had siblings at home, and they needed to be taken care of, too. But at the time, she was very lonely. Her sisters never visited her in the hospital. But her grandparents came, and brought her a stuffed dog, which she named Fido, that was to see her through that bad time and several others.

Patricia received special attention and gifts from her family when she came home, and was thoroughly spoiled during that part of her life.

When I came home [from the hospital], my sisters and everybody was all over me. And it was like party time. Then I got a brand new television set . . . a stereo. It was three in one. A television set, stereo, and radio. . . . Everyone thought I was going to die. So, I wanted a TV and a stereo, and that's what I got. I was spoiled . . . really spoiled.

Not that Patricia thinks spoiling a child is necessarily a good idea.

That causes problems with a child's behavior, too. Spoiling a child at this time can bring major problems later. Parents have to try to be cautious about spoiling a child who is sick because it would be your first instinct to do that.

Still, it wasn't a happy time. Patricia remembers seeing other children outside playing and running on the street, while she had to remain on the front porch.

My parents let me go to the front porch but that was about it. I had to be restricted and therefore my childhood remained . . . uh . . . a very protective time with little independence. I'd watch the kids go up and down the [street]. I was on the glider [porch swing] with a blanket on. I was sitting there and everybody was playing around me. And I would just be sitting there.

Her sisters tried to ease the boredom, engaging her in quiet games. "My sisters, I must say, were always good to me, though I mean . . . if I couldn't go outside, they'd play like Racko or something like card games [with me]. I didn't have much energy anyway since it was taken away, you know." But she was not allowed to participate in anything physical.

I had to be watched all the time 'cause I couldn't have a bunch of bruises all over me. I mean kids will be kids and all but I had to be careful not to have a lot of bruises. So, I was allowed outside for a little bit but not for a long time because if I fell over a branch or something there would have been bruises. I don't know . . . I got to do things but I do feel like I was restricted a lot.

Patricia thought she had a good relationship with her sisters. However, in a recent conversation with her eldest sister, she discovered how resentful at least one of them was about the attention her parents paid to her.

[My] oldest [sister] had the bedroom close[st] to the kitchen. She said they [my parents] were talking one night and she overheard them talking about me . . . about my dying. Then she said she heard them say I was their favorite kid. She said she couldn't believe that I was their favorite. And she just stood [there] and said she'd always remember that and she kind of hated me for that.

Patricia has never really resolved this issue with her sister. "I am still handling these kinds of things from so long ago. It stays with you. It follows you."

Neither Patricia nor her family was very religious.

I went to church . . . but not very often. We were Methodist. This one week I really wanted to go . . . 'cause see I knew all the books of the Bible to get my ribbons. But then . . . my dad's work shift changed . . . and we didn't go [to church] that week. I then forgot all them books . . . I never got my ribbons . . . and I [decided] I won't ever go back to church again.

But she and her family do think of her survival as a miracle from God.

My dad [told me] that he asked God if I was going to live. He was in our backyard down on his knees looking up into the sky . . . where heaven is supposed to be. He said he looked up and a yes came in the clouds. I guess my dad wasn't so tough after all. You know . . . I don't know about miracles. But maybe I am one. Kids weren't surviving this [ALL] back in 1966. Well, what can I say? I'm still here after all these years and I've survived.

Patricia's mother had another theory about why she survived. My "mom says . . . she thinks . . . when they finally let me come home . . . and I was so sick [from the measles] with the fever and everything . . . that's what really burned the leukemia out of me." Patricia herself doesn't know why she made it, when so many others didn't. "Who really knows for sure? Whether it was God in the clouds, the measles, the doctors, or me . . . I'll never really know. But I'm still here. That's what I know."

To this day, Patricia's family doesn't really discuss her leukemia or that difficult time in all their lives. But every year, one of her sisters participates in a fund-raising event held in Pittsburgh for Children's Hospital to benefit the cure for leukemia.

Every year like from K-Mart or KDKA or something they have a benefit for Children's Hospital and leukemia. And the one sister always asked me do you want a stuffed white bear or a T-shirt . . . or anything they had. You know . . . it [proceeds] goes to Children's Hospital for leukemia. Then they'll have a Jell-O slide; it's at the Hilton in downtown Pittsburgh. These people would slide down into Jell-O. And she did that for me. She got up there and they said [her name] and this is for her sister [my name] who had leukemia. And then she went down the slide into 500 pounds of Jell-O. She had to get people to sponsor her for the money. So . . . it kind of made me feel good that she would do something like that for me. When I found out my sister was doing it, I even donated money for her to do it. Even though it was for me, I gave it to her because . . . hey . . . it's not for me. It's for the cause and for the kids.

THE SCHOOL EXPERIENCE

Once she was in remission, Patricia returned to her second-grade class in the local public elementary school. "I didn't go right back to school when I came home from the hospital" but she did return before the end of the school year. All the time that she was absent and sick, she and her parents were conscientious about her keeping up with her schoolwork. "My sister would bring the work home for me. They [my parents] brought it to me in the hospital." Patricia worked on it at night, on her own. Then her sisters would take it back to school."

Before she returned to school, her mother told everyone at school about "her situation." Then as she went through the various grades, it seemed each teacher knew.

My mom let everyone know at school. The teacher and the principal knew I was sick. . . . Like I said, I had to be watched . . . like going out to recess and stuff like that. I think everyone knew the whole way through school . . . at least in the elementary years . . . but I never did . . . they managed to keep it from me . . . all them people.

Returning to school was uneventful. She had only been gone a few months.

I don't think I had been afraid to go back to school . . . 'cause I liked school. You know. It was positive compared to other things in my life at that time . . . things that hurt . . . or feeling lonely. School was a safe place . . . with friends. . . . [It was] normal. I think going to school is important and better for the kids so they wouldn't feel lonely.

Her classmates welcomed her back without fuss, and accepted her explanations of why she had been absent.

Well, one kid that I was in school with, his name was Ed. He remembers me missing a lot of school . . . and then me coming back. I sat right in front of him. And [one day] . . . he said, "Why was you gone so long?" And [I said], "Hey, 'cause I had . . . pneumonia and the measles." It was just like that.

Patricia remembers having one close friend in second grade; a neighbor child named Monica. They went all through school together.

She'd come over . . . she was never afraid of me . . . she never said anything. Monica and I used to take baths together . . . I mean when we were kids. . . . I think if they thought I was really sick . . . I think people would have run away from me. I think that's what my parents thought anyhow . . . they thought I'd be treated differently . . . or looked at differently.

And making and keeping friends was never a problem for Patricia. "I still have friends from when I was in the sixth grade. I'm still close with them . . . we've gone through different things, back and forth . . . what I've had . . . what they've had . . . isn't that friendship . . . sticking it out . . . being there for each other."

AREAS OF SCHOOL DIFFICULTY

Some of the schoolwork, even in second grade, was hard. Patricia's attendance was sporadic. "I was absent 'cause I was sick from the medicine or I had a headache. I got them headaches frequently. Maybe that's why I never got to the place the other kids were at in reading."

At the end of the school year, Patricia was promoted, with her friends, to third grade. She believes now that that was a mistake.

Yea . . . one thing I regret, I wish that I would have been retained. I feel I really lost a lot in reading. I wish I would have been held back. Maybe things would have been different for my life and me today if I could read. I am not saying they would have been but they might have been different . . . better . . . you know. They moved me onward . . . when they shouldn't have . . . as the years went by . . . everything got harder and harder for me. I was always in the low reading class. . . . I was with the [other kids] who were low in reading too . . . they didn't pull us out individually. It was just a room of us. I think I was in this low reading class until 10th grade.

Not all subjects were hard for her. "I always got Ds in reading and As in math . . . I'm good at math. I love abstract reasoning and puzzles. I took difficult math classes like Algebra I and II, Calculus . . . because I really wanted to work with numbers." Spelling was a little difficult for her. "There are a lot of words that I can pronounce but I can't spell them." And writing required at least one revision. "I always have it on scratch [paper], then do it on good [paper]. I . . . do it twice always. I don't ever . . . just sit down . . . and just write. Telling a story I could do . . . but I always had to work it out first on another sheet of paper."

But Patricia's reading problems were the biggest obstacle to school success. "As far as like reading . . . to comprehend, I'm really bad." School was a tremendous struggle because of her reading difficulties.

I remember if teachers made stuff interesting, it was much better for me. [There was a class called] World Cultures. I thought I'd hate World Cultures. But my teacher was excellent. I mean, at the time, I knew about world cultures because of the teacher. It wasn't a boring thing to him. He was into it. When you have something like that, you listen and learn instead of just reading the stuff.

And she had to work very hard, just to get through.

I did my best . . . I mean I tried and I tried. Then I thought they might flunk me in my senior year. . . . I said forget this . . . I ain't staying in school no more. I really cracked down and tried to study . . . but it still hurts that it was my best . . . and all I ever got was a D.

To this day, reading is still a problem for her. To understand what she is reading takes her total concentration. If there is the slightest distraction, she is lost.

I read the newspaper every once in awhile. . . . But, I mean, only if something catches my eye on the first page. I can't deal with people talking to me when I'm trying to . . . concentrate. It's like I pick up the newspaper and I'll read the front page or something, and [if somebody will say something to me . . . [whatever it was . . . it went right out the door . . . and I have to start all over again. As long as they talk . . . whatever I read . . . I'll forget it.

She has developed some compensatory strategies.

I go to another room and read it . . . to figure out what I'm trying to read, but if anything is going on like the TV or the teakettle going off . . . I'm lost. . . . I can do anything you tell me to do . . . or you show me to do. But if you make me read, I can't do anything. It limits my life and my dreams.

At one time, Patricia wanted to be an accountant "because I love figures" but her reading problems stood in her way. "I don't like to read. Reading brings me misery. Reading is everything."

As an adult, Patricia decided to enroll in an adult education class.

I was working midnight on my job, I thought I'm going to school during the day. So I went to commercial school. They had a reading course that you had to go through. Anyway, you had to do [all the work] in class. I mean the book did not leave the class. You had to do it there and turn it in to the teacher. Well, when everybody got assigned their reading things, the reading levels went from A to K. Everybody was in F or G. I wasn't. I was in C. I mean I know I should have been in level F but I was like in three lower levels than everybody else was in the entire classroom. I was 28 at the time.

But the class didn't work out. She couldn't concentrate with all the students in the classroom talking and causing distractions.

When the teacher would leave the classroom, and I'd be like reading, then everybody would start talking. That would just blow me out of what I had just read. They would just be talking among themselves, and my concentration would go right out the window. And it was like . . . I can't do this. I need to have quiet to understand what I'm doing. So I lasted only 3 weeks. They offered daylight at work. I told them I had quit [the class]. They said, "Why did you quit?" I said, "Hey, they offered me daylight." The truth is it was so embarrassing to me.

SURVIVING

Patricia talks quietly about her childhood experience of having ALL, but "I can turn real emotional in a minute over the whole ordeal." There are several ways in which Patricia believes the cancer experience has impacted her life. "It makes up a part of who you are today and where you are today. That time period definitely impacts your life. I learned about pain . . . fear . . . and loneliness as a child." Furthermore, the cancer took away her childhood.

When a child goes through this, they grow up quickly, and mature more quickly than other children. Part of my childhood was taken away and that's something you can't ever get back. I can't go back and get it back. It's over. Some things are gone forever. What's the word? Finite. Your childhood helps to form you into being an adult. I missed part of my childhood, so maybe something is missing in my adult life now. I feel as if something is incomplete now . . . in my adulthood. Like I missed a step or something on life's developmental ladder. I feel like an incomplete adult because I had an incomplete childhood . . . I didn't get to be just a kid . . . you know? I suppose that sounds weird and wouldn't a psychologist have a field day with that one.

It left her with reading difficulties she has not been able to overcome.

I can read but I am not very good at it. I wish I would have been held back in school. I now know that all I am ever going to be is what I am . . . a factory worker because I can't read well. My future ends here. If you can read, then you can have a bigger and brighter future. You could be anything you wanted to be and have a choice of jobs as well as a higher income. You could have a nice home and maybe travel but . . . for me . . . this is it because I don't read well. My life will be limited. My dream of reading better went out the window when I quit the reading class. I know that. But I couldn't do the work in class. I had to choose . . . or maybe I had no choice when it came down to it. Anyway, I left the class and I left my future there too. So . . . that's it for learning to read . . . that's it for my future too.

Recurrence is a constant worry, somewhere far in the back of her mind.

I mean, it never actually leaves you . . . ever. 'Cause it's like it will always be there. Not that it is always on your mind . . . but it's always there. You know? Like when I got that cancer of the cervix, I thought . . . oh no. Here it comes. It's coming back and . . . I started freaking out. I mean it was for nothing . . . it was done . . . over with . . . done. They say it's in remission. I think to myself sometimes . . . is this going to be a lifetime for me . . . or . . . is it not? Nobody knows. Nobody does. I go do a lot of things and never worry about it. But . . . it is always there.

And she is still struggling to understand why her parents never told her she had leukemia, and whether not knowing made her into a liar.

I'm glad I know what was wrong with everything and me. My grandparents and the neighbors knew, but I didn't. It is interesting that it never crossed over all those years with other family members knowing. I thought, "How could you do that to me?" I am not a person that lies . . . you know? . . . I still, once in awhile, will get angry over it. I'll say, "I still don't know why you didn't tell me the truth?" But then I'll let it drop; you know, why dwell on things? But it's irritating . . . they didn't say anything. Things just don't go away like that.

Despite the negatives, Patricia believes the cancer experience helped shape her, positively, into the adult she is today.

It did make me a survivor and I have survived things that I shouldn't have. So, I know I am supposed to be here. Well, maybe everything isn't perfect. . . . I can't read well . . . and I don't have the greatest job . . . and I don't have a lot of money . . . and I can't travel around the world. But I am alive. I can enjoy a beautiful day, a sunset, and a good dinner. I can enjoy and love my family and friends. I can have fun and laugh. It's the simple things in life that give you great possibilities. My life isn't perfect. But then, who really does have a perfect life?

The cancer experience also brought out some very positive values in her parents. She described them in relation to her family's reaction to her losing her hair.

Dying is more tragic than losing your hair in trying not to die. So . . . you live with no hair for a time . . . big deal. It seems like a small price to pay so you can live to be an adult. Men go around with bald heads all the time. Is anything said to them? It's just a fact of life that most men become bald. It's accepted and you go on. I've never heard of a woman divorcing her husband because his physical appearance is changed from when they were married by becoming bald. You love the person not the hair. So . . . I guess I was loved and my not having hair just didn't matter at the time. Hopefully, people are deeper than that and can see past human . . . what is it . . . human vulnerabilities or frailties. If someone can't, then they ain't worth being around.

The cancer experience also provided Patricia with a good luck charm, the stuffed animal her grandparents had given her.

Do you know I kept that stuffed dog . . . for myself? In fact, I had a back operation last October [and] I pulled it back out. It must have some significance with me [around] survival. Pretty deep, huh? It is funny how we relate to things in an odd sorta way. So I took it out and just set it on top of my stand at the hospital. I took it out when I had the cervical cancer, too. It was inside my hope chest. Maybe it's for comfort. It's still on top of my stand at home now. Its name is Fido. Well, it's pretty ratty now, but I just can't part with it . . . I suppose the danger of malignancy can be more than just physical; it goes into your psyche as well. I just can't say good-bye to that stuffed dog. It means survival to me in more ways than one.

Patricia would like to marry, and have children.

If I ever got married, I'd have to tell my husband because there is a chance it might come in our kids. [There's] a chance the kids might be deformed [because of the treatment]. They are really not sure if I'd ever reproduce because treatments do affect those kinds of things. I could have a perfectly normal baby, but then I may not. And that would have to be the chance that my husband and me would have to take.

And she is optimistic about the future. She hopes her job at the printshop will continue.

I like my job. Today, I work on computers in the bindery . . . and I can do that. I mean, I can tell you, and I'm not bragging, but I am pretty good at my job. A lot of people, unfortunately, are not in jobs they like and enjoy, and it affects other parts of their lives. That's what I am afraid of, if I have to get a new job.

She believes she has a purpose on this earth.

All I can say is my life has been pretty good so far. This [life] is all temporary anyway. So, if you get a second chance, like I did, to stay on this earth a bit longer, you owe it to yourself to be good to yourself, to accept yourself, to do those things that make you happy, and to love . . . because it will end one day. I know that my experiences with cancer as a child and as an adult have caused me to have a "different life" and to be a "different person." It would be good to one day look back at my life and think, boy . . . my life made a difference because I was given a different life.

And she considers herself both a pioneer in leukemia and a miracle for having survived during a time when survival was almost nonexistent for childhood leukemia patients.

I really wish there were a cure for it so that people wouldn't have to go through it. It changes so many lives. These children go through so much. When I say something to people about [having leukemia as a child], they say how did you survive it? I say, "Hey, I'm here!" Some people say it is a miracle I am here . . . yes . . . I am a miracle.

4

Giving My All!

Elaine's Story

If you want to get more out of life, you have to give more to life.

—John Marks Templeton

Elaine is 25 years old, 5'7" tall, with blond hair. She is the youngest in her family; she has one brother, 10 years her senior. She lives in a moderate-sized town southwest of Pittsburgh and works as a pediatric nurse. She has been a nurse for 5 years. She is attractive with a bubbly personality. Elaine was quite enthusiastic about sharing her thoughts and feelings. "No one had ever asked me from the hospital or school what the experience was really like," she said. She looked forward to being able to discuss her experience at last and, hopefully, to help others going through a similar experience.

ONSET OF THE DISEASE AND TREATMENT

In November 1975, Elaine was experiencing swelling of her lymph nodes.

I was 6 years old and it started around Thanksgiving. My parents didn't know what it was. They thought maybe I had the mumps. I remember we had gone out for a big Thanksgiving dinner, the whole family. I was dressed up in a little bonnet and a long dress and stuff.

Everyone was like, gosh, her neck is so big. A little while later, they took me to our family doctor in Wheeling, West Virginia. She knew immediately after doing some tests that it wasn't the mumps. So, after that, I came to Children's Hospital in Pittsburgh. There I had a biopsy of my neck done.

Elaine was first admitted to Children's Hospital of Pittsburgh on December 5, 1975, with fatigue, pain in her ear, and cervical bilateral adenopathy. After performing biopsies to the lung, the right lymph node of the neck, and the bone marrow, Elaine was diagnosed on December 7 with lymphosarcoma (indistinguishable from ALL and is treated exactly the same as ALL). With this desease, there is more bone marrow and lymph node involvement but it is a cancer of blood-forming tissue. She was 6 years old, and in the first grade. Her treatment regime began immediately and lasted for 12 days. She received prednisone, vincrinstine, L-asparaginase, cytoxan, and intrathecal methotrexate. Radiation of 2,400 cGx was administered to the brain and neck from February 12 through March 4, 1976; she had 16 treatments in 21 days. Elaine was discharged on December 19, 1975, still receiving chemotherapy at home and on weekly visits to the hospital.

Elaine was in and out of the hospital between November 1975 and May 1976. For example, she was discharged on December 19 but had to return just before Christmas. Her memories of this time are vivid.

It was Christmastime. I had a collapsed lung at home. We went to the doctor's office and they took one look at my eyes and said, "Oh my gosh, get her over to Children's." I was in septic shock. Septic shock is when your immune system is so low, then you become septic. You don't have an immune system. I got a staph infection in all my vital organs . . . my liver . . . my kidneys . . . my lungs . . . all through my body. I was in shock, which meant I needed fluids. All my veins had collapsed. What happens is you can't see all the little veins because there is no fluid. You are dehydrated; your blood is not profusing through your body. And you're not profusing oxygen. So, they had to do what is called "cut-downs." They had to cut my skin and go down underneath where they can find the veins. And they pull the veins up. That's how they get the IVs in you.

As for the collapsed lung,

I remember them putting my chest tube in. When they did that, I was in intensive care for 3 days. That's when I lost my hair. They put a chest tube in to get the fluid out through the tube. I remember every day the lungs reinflating.

That hospital stay lasted from December to February. Then, from February through April, she was in and out with various types of infections and setbacks. When not admitted, she would come to Children's three times per week for her chemotherapy and checkups. By January 9, 1976, there were signs of muscle atrophy due to the disease. "I was in a wheelchair. I can remember my parents trying to teach me to walk at home. I couldn't walk. They would try to hold on to me to get me to walk up the steps."

In March 1976, she was admitted with a high fever, severe diarrhea, alopecia, pneumonia, and methotrexate toxicity. She was admitted again at Eastertime, from April 19, 1976, to May 9, 1976, for a lung biopsy that revealed pneumosystis pneumonia.

. . . a rare form of pneumonia. It's that kind of pneumonia that the AIDs people get . . . usually right before they die. It was then that they stopped my chemotherapy altogether.

Soon, the doctors started her back on chemotherapy, 6-MP and methotrexate. But just before her discharge, she was exposed to chicken pox by a girl who had come into her room at the hospital.

And, of course, I wasn't allowed to get them. So, they gave me some medication to stop them so you can't get them. I remember that was sort of a devastating thing,'cause I wasn't allowed to go home. Then they had to give all kinds of stuff because I had a reaction to the drip. They had to give me benadryl and something else because I had an allergic reaction.

Elaine was finally discharged on the day before her birthday, May 10, in time for a birthday party at home.

Throughout that next summer, Elaine's parents tried to give her a normal, happy life.

My parents did really well not being overly protective of me. Actually that year that I got out of the hospital, you know, in May, I went to the beach three times. My aunt, my mom's sister, scared my mom to death. Thank goodness my dad wasn't there at the time, because he probably would have had a conniption. She [my aunt] had me out on a raft all the way out in the ocean and I fell off once and went tumbling.

Elaine continued to receive chemotherapy until about age 10 (fourth grade). Treatments ended almost exactly 4 years from the time of her initial diagnosis. During those years, she continued to receive methotrexate and 6-MP, orally, and an intramuscular shot of vincrinstine, once a month. Elaine continued to go to Children's for her annual checkups and has had no anti-cancer medications administered to her since the day the chemotherapy had been stopped. There has been no recurrence of the disease either in its primary state or in any secondary forms of cancer.

ELAINE'S REACTIONS TO DIAGNOSIS AND TREATMENT

At the time of her initial diagnosis and treatment, Elaine was not really aware that she was fighting a very serious battle against cancer. Her parents and doctors never actually sat down and told her exactly what the disease was that had caused her to be so gravely ill. Yet, Elaine doesn't remember not having been told, since she feels she always suspected that she had cancer. It is only recently that her parents confirmed that it had taken 2 or 3 years for them to tell her.

I thought I knew. Here . . . I thought I knew the whole time that I had cancer. But I just found out like last week that actually I really didn't. I guess I was 6 when [I was] diagnosed but I wasn't told that I had cancer until I was 8 or 9. I've always told people, through the years, that I always knew I had cancer. But all I really knew was I was a sick little girl. I knew what was going on around me because I was really smart, too. But I just didn't know what cancer was; at 6, you don't really comprehend what cancer is.

Elaine handled the hospital procedures very well, but they were painful and memorable.

They gave you spinal taps and bone marrows all the time . . . lots and lots. And whenever they would give me my chemo, I would have it put in the spine. I was awake for all of them. The ones that stick out most are the most recent ones. I was probably 17 and I had to have a bone marrow and spinal tap. It really was a painful experience. And just this past weekend, I took a class called "pediatric exam life support." During this class, we learned how to put in a certain kind of IV. I saw this needle and I thought, "Oh my God." It sort of made me sick . . . because I hadn't seen it since my last bone marrow. And I thought, "Oh my gosh . . . I've had that put in me." It almost looks like a nail. As soon as I saw it, it brought back [memories]. . . . My whole time being a nurse, in the past 5 years . . . nothing has made me sick. Nothing has ever bothered me . . . nothing . . . and when I saw that just last week, that really bothered me bad . . . it was a really painful experience.

Even the oral medications were "difficult to swallow."

Prednisone is very, very bitter . . . it is a horrible, horrible bitter taste. [The nurse] took my prednisone and crushed it and put it on a spoon with water, like you do baby aspirin. And she made me take it that way. And after that, I wouldn't put anything into my mouth. They had the hardest time getting me to take my medicine after that. Then my mom started putting all my meds into gelatin capsules so you can't taste the pills, and they go down easily. But I remember that horrible awful taste.

Elaine also had a bad experience with one particular technician who came to draw blood, and with one particular nurse assigned to her.

Every day they would come in and take blood out of your finger. You know, I wouldn't have any problems with people drawing blood or anything. One day this lady came in and she had greasy, grimy hair and stuff. And she took the lance and put it in my finger and twisted it. After that, I didn't want anyone coming near me. My mom would never let that lady ever come back in my room. I think there was one [nurse] that I really didn't like because she was so bossy with me. I think she wanted me to be a little older than I was. She would get upset when I wanted my mom . . . you know, just bossy.

Hospital rules and restrictions were frustrating to the 6-year-old.

It was around Eastertime. I used to get not only candy but I used to get all kinds of toys in the Easter basket. Well, one of my favorite things was this plastic bubble blow stuff. It had a little tube, and you blew it out. It smelled really bad. And here I was with this horrible pneumonia. I could hardly breathe. I was like gasping for every breath, but I wanted this blow stuff because I wanted to blow it so bad. And they wouldn't let me do it because my lungs were so bad, and because of the smell. To this day, it still upsets me that they wouldn't let me have that bubble blow stuff. You know, the one thing I wanted. And I thought, "Mom, why don't you just let me have it?" That was the one thing that would have made me happy.

But, most of the time, Elaine had a very positive attitude about what she was going through and was treated very well.

I remember really good things about my doctors. I had one that was really special to me. He was a resident at the time. I called him Dr. Dave. Whenever other doctors couldn't get IVs in they would always call him and he would come in. He was really special. He was just a wonderful person. He used to come in with Rocky and Bullwinkle and play it . . . hand puppets and stuff. He was really a special guy. We used to have squirt gun battles and things in the hospital. You know . . . for a doctor to be like that . . . that was really neat . . . because it meant a lot to me. Kids get attached to their doctors. Oh, I was definitely attached.

Elaine also remembers the nurses.

The nurses were pretty much wonderful. I had a nurse, also, that was really, really special to me. Her name was Marilyn. I was always really creative, even when I was 6. I always did all kinds of creative things. And I made little paper flowers for her [Marilyn's] wedding when she got married. I made all the flowers for their cars out of tissue paper. So, that was really neat. And when I left the hospital, she gave me a little present . . . for Christmas that year. She gave me a daisy for the Christmas tree. I still have my daisy. It's like a really pretty glass daisy for the Christmas tree and I still have it. And she gave me a little water bottle. It was a little elephant water bottle.

And there were even some good times.

[On] Christmas [day] I was in my own room because I remember getting my Christmas presents. I remember one of the things was this Indian bead maker, that I made necklaces [with]. And since then, I have always been a jewelry person. I had all kinds of presents but I was too sick to enjoy any of them. But I do recall the necklace and earring maker. Also, the hospital has Sesame Street *characters there and football players for Christmas. I recall there was a Christmas tree and a party. My doctor, Dr. Dave, played the piano.*

TREATMENT SIDE EFFECTS

Elaine experienced some mild and transient side effects of the treatments she received.

I don't remember throwing up. I used to get diarrhea really, really bad. I can remember them giving me this little doughnut to sit on, a little rubber doughnut because my little bottom was so sore.

Elaine was "chubby while I was on prednisone. That makes you swell. Then when the prednisone stopped I was like a little stick and everyone was trying to get me to eat." But the most devastating side effect was hair loss—or at least the anticipation of hair loss. When she finally lost her hair, she was so sick that it didn't even matter.

I was in ICU in December that's when I lost my hair. No matter how many times they poked me . . . or did anything . . . no matter what, I had long blond hair all the way down my back. I wore it long all the time. I knew I was going to lose my hair and it was one of the hardest things. When I did finally lose it . . . then it didn't even matter because I so sick. But it all came off.

Elaine also used to get severe migraine headaches.

I couldn't go to school. All the lights would have to be out. I'd have to lie on the floor in complete darkness. I couldn't move my head. Those migraines lasted 10 years until the 9th or 10th grade.

Elaine has learned to live with several long-term side effects, as well.

I have a big indentation in my leg. It looks something like a huge dimple, from where the needle hit the nerves. I do have my right arm a little weaker than my left arm because that is where my chest tube was when my lung collapsed. And to this day, my one side is a little bit lower than the other side. And you know, just this year, I had x-rays done and the doctor pointed out to me that my spine is crooked.

But what are hardest for her are the scars on her body, constant reminders of the cancer.

I had gallstones that had to be operated on. I didn't have to have a horrible surgery but I had a colon sysectomy. That was something that really bothered me because of all the scars all over my body from the cancer. My belly was the only place I didn't have scars and that was sort of like my sanctuary. That was my one place. My sexy place on my body. Then they told me they would have to operate there. It really upset me. And now I have scars there, too.

After all these years, Elaine is experiencing a kind of posttraumatic stress syndrome, perhaps similar to soldiers of war. She is noticing extreme anxiety and she is developing "cancer paranoia" when she is not feeling well.

When I had the gallstones problem, I thought, "Oh no, I am really sick again." I am thinking of seeing a counselor. I mean, I don't have any problems telling you that. I tell people at work that I think I am going to go. I have high anxiety now. It is not all the time . . . it just gets to be overwhelming. I am ready to look directly at the problem.

She is also worried about sterility.

I have asked about that all through the years because it has meant a lot to me . . . to have babies. I've never had any problems. I have always been very regular . . . my menstrual period . . . menstrual cycle. And hopefully some day I will be able to have a baby. I have no irregularities that I know of.

IMPACT ON THE FAMILY

My family was really supportive. My mom was with me all the time. [She] stayed at Children's with me. And my dad worked. It was wonderful that my mom didn't work at the time so she got to be with me. You know, she stayed with me the whole time. She stayed on a cot in the room with me the entire time. I didn't even let her out of my sight, which I know was really hard on her. My dad would come up evenings and also on weekends. My dad would always bring me food. I always wanted Long John Silvers. So, he brought it to me every weekend, every night, or whenever I wanted it.

Throughout the course of her illness and treatment, Elaine's parents continued to provide support and care.

After I was out of the hospital, I was really afraid I was going to die. And I couldn't sleep; I wouldn't sleep at night. It was awful. My mom helped me a lot. I think probably until I was 10 years old, I slept in my parents' room . . . in bed . . . in their room. My mom would sleep with me because I couldn't sleep by myself . . . just for fear I was going to die. I was just really scared. And my mom used to tell me different things every night, to count. I used to count things every single night, like butterflies or something . . . some really pretty things. I don't remember dreaming bad dreams. I do remember having the scary feeling of going to sleep . . . because I was afraid I was going to die in my sleep. Oh my gosh, both my parents are wonderful people.

Elaine's parents never let her know how difficult the experience was for them.

I don't remember ever seeing my mother cry . . . what a strain it must have been on them . . . more on my mom. Now they talk that they didn't want me to see how it was. They wanted everything to be good for me.

And although psychological services were not available at the hospital, Elaine's parents found ways to cope.

I know that my mom after I was out of the hospital, finally, she went to like, not a rehab, but a psychiatric place for awhile. After I was home, just for a rest. Just to get away for awhile . . . from me. So, I went and stayed with my aunt when my mother went to that place. I think it was like 2 or 3 weeks. My mom didn't tell me at the time what she was doing . . . what happened.

Elaine, too, found ways to cope. She never had an imaginary friend or stuffed animals to cling to; she fell back on her creativity.

The thing I absolutely loved to do was color. If something bothered me or if I was really, really upset about something . . . I'd go in my room to color. And it took all the stress and strain. The coloring meant something to me. It's one of my favorite things to do . . . from when I was very young until now. I still have my big huge box of crayons . . . I think the coloring helped a lot. I was always drawing pictures and doing crafty things. I was good using my hands and teaching other people . . . that was another thing that helped me . . . that I was usually the one helping other people.

There were no grandparents to help, but aunts, uncles, and cousins offered their support from time to time.

Aunts and uncles would come visit. My cousin, Cassandra, is really a special person in my life. I was always like her little girl. She would take me to do things and come and see me all the time.

Sadly, however, Elaine's relationship with her older brother who was 16–17 years old during the period of her diagnosis and treatment was forever altered by her disease.

It was really hard on him, I think. He didn't visit me a whole lot. He's had a lot of problems over the years. I think it stems back to when I was sick. He got really rebellious after that, for attention from my parents. After my parents were with me, he had an attitude of, well, you weren't there for me, Why should I do what you say? Whenever he would come to visit, I would love it, because he meant the world to me. But, I remember he didn't come very much. I think it really scared him.

THE SCHOOL EXPERIENCE

Elaine missed most of first grade, from the middle of November 1975 through June 1976. She had a hospital tutor at Children's Hospital while she was being treated and on subsequent visits when she was admitted for an extended stay she attended a hospital school. "I would go down and to class or whatever. You could attend when you were feeling well enough. But usually I couldn't." Education was important in her life.

I remember them bringing my schoolwork when I first wasn't real sick. My friends would bring the work home and my parents would try to teach me. But then, I was in the hospital so much and I think they had a tutor at the hospital that would come up in the room and tutor me. The tutor at the hospital could be your tutor outside of the hospital too. And she probably talked to my teacher at my school. It was sort of hard because I was from a different state [her school was in West Virginia while she was being treated in Pennsylvania].

When she returned home in May, Elaine had a home tutor for the final month of the school year.

I remember this man would come to the house and tutor me at home. I think it was once or twice a week . . . he would come to my home for like 4 or 5 hours. [Then,] I just went right on into the second grade. I was a really smart little girl. They tested me and I was in the top 10 percentile. It was a pretty good transition back to school. I got to start right at the beginning of the year.

Second and third grades were uneventful. Elaine missed very little school even though she was on a maintenance regime that involved oral medications, shots, and a monthly visit to the hospital.

But then in fourth grade, I had to leave because of a chicken pox outbreak. That was really hard because I was all better. I was considered cured by fourth grade . . . and then the chicken pox. I always knew I had to be real careful about getting around kids who had chicken pox. I suppose it wasn't really a bad thing. I missed all of fourth grade. I had a homebound teacher that used to come to the house. The homebound people were really nice. She would come twice a week and she used to take me out, too. We would go do things . . . go to the park, and go see movies. After I had my studies, then we would go.

Elaine's parents were determined to maintain her in some form of education at all times. "That's how I got the tutors and also homebound teachers." Her mother took on the responsibility of informing teachers of her illness, treatment, and progress. Both parents helped her with her schoolwork.

I was always at the top of my reading class. My parents had a lot to do with it. My mother would go and talk to my teachers and sometimes would get my assignments and sometimes the tutor would get my assignments. But my parents also taught me. I mean they read to me all the time. And I read to them. They would always do math with me like writing me multiplication problems. I remember my mother taking out pieces of her checkbook and writing down number problems and I would do all of them. I remember them playing games with me.

Elaine had a special relationship with most teachers.

I was sort of special to my teachers [after coming back to school]. I used to, at times, play into my illness. I would say, "I don't want go out and play." Then, I would stay in and grade papers with the teachers a lot of the times. My second-grade teacher was really good. She used to come [visit me at the hospital]. I was like her special girl. She used to do all kinds of special things for me.

   I remember I had another special relationship with [my third-grade teacher]. I got to be really close to [the homebound teacher] and her family. I would go up to her house.

And she was disappointed when her teachers did not take a special interest in her.

I remember my first-grade teacher never came and saw me [at the hospital]. It was like she didn't care. She was just sort of weird. My fourth-grade teacher was not mean but I think she had some animosity. I think it made her upset that I didn't go to school because I was a good student. Then when I did go back to school, she was standoffish.

By junior high and high school, Elaine also developed close relationships with the guidance counselors.

I've always talked to my teachers and counselors. Junior high was great because then I had counselors to talk to frequently. They all knew what my problems were. Especially, this one in ninth grade. She became a good friend and I used to baby-sit for her and her family. I remember talking to her about my menstrual cycles because I started worrying about, you know, whether I was going to be normal . . . whether things were going to be different than like other girls.

Academically, school was fine, but Elaine had some difficulties with her peers.

Most of the kids that I went to school with were around my community, too. And a lot of them sort of knew I was sick. I had to explain to them what was going on with me. It was really hard on friends. They really didn't understand. They just knew I was really sick.

I did have a couple of kids tease me, but I think it was not knowing that made them tease me. I think that is what makes kids tease other kids. They don't know what's going on and they are more unsure of themselves. They tease other kids because they don't know what's going on. And, when someone is different, of course, they are going to tease.

When Elaine returned to school in second grade, she still didn't have any hair.

I used to wear a scarf all the time. I wasn't a wig girl. I wore scarves that matched all my little outfits. I always had friends . . . a lot of friends even though I was going in and out of the program. They knew who I was, and they knew what kind of person I was. And I was always nice to everyone and I don't think they really cared what it was under that scarf. But I remember one of the kids teasing me. He'd say, "What's under there? What's under there?" Then, one time that little boy did try to pull my scarf off. I think that really bothered me. My brother used to tease me, too. He'd call me egghead.

Missing fourth grade was also hard on Elaine "because of friends."

I remember my best friend [what is really neat is she is still my best friend). I met her in fourth grade when the chicken pox outbreak happened. It was the beginning of the year; she had transferred from another school. Over the years, she has told me, "You were the only person who was nice to me. Then you left." She said she didn't understand when I had to leave . . . what was wrong.

And throughout school, Elaine "had a lot of problems in school with how kids treated me because they were jealous of me."

In seventh or eighth grade, a girl almost beat me up. The students would recognize I was special and that has made kids jealous of me my whole life, because of the attention that it brought. Even in junior high, in the seventh grade, I had problems with other kids because I seem to be the kind of person that attracts people. And people have a really hard time dealing with that. It's the type of person I am.

Elaine was never retained despite missing nearly two full grade levels of school. She believes that had she been, she would have felt "devastated. I think it would have been really hard. I might have understood later on but not then. I had a friend who had leukemia and he got held back because of it. But I wish they hadn't."

At age 19, when Elaine was in nursing school, she finally contracted chicken pox. Nearly 15 years after being diagnosed with cancer, her fears returned.

I missed a whole month of nursing school because of chicken pox. It was a really scary time because I was told you couldn't get the chicken pox. I was really, really scared. I went to the emergency room . . . it was horrible . . . it was devastating. I was deathly, deathly ill. I had a real high fever. And I was very, very anxious and scared so the doctor gave me something for the anxiety. Here my immunity system must have gone down, even after all those years, and I was exposed to a student in clinicals. It was one of the worst experiences of my adult life.

Nevertheless, Elaine's innate academic ability got her through, with a little help from her friends.

My classmates were wonderful. They took notes for me and brought them home for me. The teachers were wonderful. I don't even know how I passed nursing school after missing a whole month. Missing a month of nursing school is like missing a year. I kept up with my work. The teachers let me take tests after I got better.

AREAS OF SCHOOL DIFFICULTY

Elaine was always considered an exceptional student. She was really good in spelling and would win all the spelling bees. She did very well in reading. She never had any difficulties in reading. Elaine viewed herself as highly proficient and actually excelled in reading.

I was always a perfectionist, too. I wanted everything to be perfect. And when things weren't I got really upset. And my parents were never ones that said you had to get straight As. They were never like that. I did it to myself. I used to cry if I didn't get As. It would be horrible. *My mom would say to me, "What am I going to do with you?" She was like "Hon, it doesn't matter. You can fail."*

Throughout elementary school, she had been recommended by her teachers for the gifted and talented program. But on the IQ test administered to determine eligibility, her verbal scores were high, but the performance scores were low.

I got straight As. I was always at the top of my class. All my other friends were in the gifted and talented class, but I wasn't. They would give me those tests and they would really frustrate me because it was more of like puzzle kinds of things you had to do. And I could never pass one of those tests. That is something that really bothered me because all my friends were in there. Even though I was an exceptional student, not being able to do that really bothered me. Why couldn't I get in the program? Here I was smart, too. I was the one getting the awards. But because each year I couldn't pass what they were measuring such as pattern things, finding things, story problems, and sequencing things, [I couldn't get into the program]. It really frustrated me. May be it had to do with problems in eye-hand coordination or something."

In fact, Elaine had severe nonverbal learning problems, and difficulties related to visual-spatial skills.

I remember now having had problems learning how to tell time. That was the hardest thing for me. In math, by fifth grade, I had a real hard time doing long division problems and story problems. By 10th grade, at age 15 or so, I had problems keeping my attention span on my work . . . like attention deficit disorder. Maybe it was because I was smart or maybe my illness and the treatment had something to do with it.

SURVIVING

There is no question that the disease, its treatment, and the aftermath have had a profound effect on Elaine's personality and outlook on life. In some ways, her innate personality shaped her response to the experience.

I sort of made the doctors happy. They would come into my room because I was such a positive little girl. They were like, gosh, how can this little girl be like this . . . when she is so sick. They told me that now that I am grown up. No matter what they did to me, it just seemed like I was never negative about it.

I think that no matter what, you should have a positive attitude about things. No matter how negative things get, there is always someone out there that's worse off than you are. That is something that has kept me going.

I am an optimist. I believe that no matter how old you are you should always have a positive attitude because look at me. I was given 3 months to live. And look, I am sitting here today.

I've seen it happen in the past 5 years of my nursing, that you can't second-guess. Anything can happen. I've seen children that were supposed to be brain dead and they've come back. Keep that positive attitude because there is a chance.

But in other ways, the experience itself has changed her, forever.

I spent a lot of time with adults. My parents never would leave me at home. I used to go all the time, with them, like to dinner or something. I did a lot of things with them. We had a family that did things together so I was exposed to many things and it really helped me. Maybe that is why I am so extroverted and social now.

I have such a bubbly personality and I get along so well with everyone. Everyone thinks like what kind of life does she have that she is so happy. It is because I had a second chance and people don't understand that.

And Elaine feels no shame about the cancer. Incredibly, she thinks of it as having been a very positive experience.

I have been telling people about my illness my whole life. I mean . . . it's always been a real positive thing. I love talking about it. And it helps so many people.

I think it's the reason I'm a nurse today. I've always wanted to do something in the medical field, since I was little, because I can give so much to other people that have this illness. Sometimes I think to myself, gosh, this person is really messing up their life by doing things like drugs or something. I wish that, just for a day, they could go through what I went through, because they would appreciate life so much more. Having the cancer made me such a better person, a stronger person. I mean if I want something I work so hard getting it, because there was a chance I might never have been able to do anything. It really has made me who I am.

It's neat what I have learned over the years. I got an advanced class that taught me a lot about life. I'm always teaching, too. I'm teaching parents and kids about their illness.

Elaine still has some problems with relationships.

My boyfriend and I just broke up. It lasted 6 months. My problem is I am very giving, sometimes too much. That bothers other people. I give all the time and I overwhelm them because they feel they can't reciprocate. It's really hard on people. I think that's what happens in my relationships with guys. My need to give and help has put me in some bad situations. I'm usually looking for someone who has problems. I ask myself, why don't I date a normal person?

I love to do special things for people. I get really upset if I don't have someone to give to. It sounds like a funny or weird problem to have. I get anxious if I don't have someone to do things for. Maybe doing things causes me to get affection and attention but I get most of my happiness out of giving things. I think that's why I am a pediatric nurse. Kids appreciate things so much and I know little things to do for them. Poor little kids . . . their bottoms get so sore and red. I know this because that was me.

And she is struggling with the reality of being a survivor.

I was given 3 months to live. The doctor told my mom it is sort of like a gate. There can be one child that gets the same exact medicines and treatments that this child gets . . . but one child breaks through the gate and makes it. There really isn't anything that says who does or doesn't. I think, why me? Why was it me who made it? I know there is some reason why I'm here. I really think it has something to do with my nursing and what I give to other kids. I know there is definitely a reason because if not I wouldn't be here . . . especially when I was only suppose to live 3 months. My mom talked about a little boy who had the same thing I had but he was never in the hospital and I was always sick in the hospital. I mean, I'd have to go in the [hospital with complications] and he never would have to go. His name was Jimmy and he ended up dying. And when I was in intensive care, I mean on death's door . . . something worked . . . something just worked. Someone above is watching over me, I know.

To deal with her feelings about survival Elaine has been thinking about "going to see a counselor." Talking to someone might also help her with her "real high anxiety [about getting sick again]. They call it 'cancer paranoia,' I think once you've had it, then you think every little [thing is cancer]. . . . I think [this anxiety] had to stem back to my illness, my childhood illness."

Elaine wants to be a pediatric nurse practitioner in an oncology unit in a children's hospital. "In Morgantown, we have Children's Hospital, but it doesn't have a floor of kids that have oncology problems." She also wants to continue her work with the Make-A-Wish Foundation.

I do a lot of things with kids, but Make-A Wish is one of the big things. They didn't have the Make-A-Wish Foundation when I was sick in 1976. That would have been something I would have absolutely loved.

And in truth, Elaine "love[s] everything. There is hardly anything I don't like in the world. I think that also stems back to my illness. I appreciate things, but most especially I appreciate my second chance at being given a life."

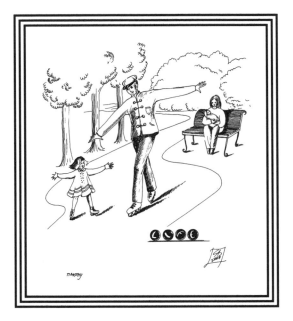

Timothy's Survival Shadow Follows Him Down the Path of Life

5

Me and My Shadow

Timothy's Story

Never fear shadows. They simply mean there's
light shining somewhere nearby.

—Ruth Renkel

Timothy is 26 years old. He has long dark tousled hair, a slim build, and is
about average height (5'6" to 5'8"). He has been married for 5 years, and
has a 4-year-old daughter as well as a newborn son. He lives in a very
small town north of Pittsburgh and works with his father in remodeling.
Timothy is the oldest child in a family of three sons. His demeanor was
very easygoing and relaxed. He commented that he had not talked about
his childhood illness in quite some time, but that he was really glad to be
called on to help. Timothy appeared very interested in the interview; several times during the discussion, he would lean back in his chair to con-
template his recollections of the various segments of his story. He spoke
with calmness and steadiness.

ONSET OF THE DISEASE AND TREATMENT

Timothy had been taken to a local hospital in the fall of 1974 with
symptoms of a cough, fever, and anemia. "I was approximately 5, turning 6. They thought I just had pneumonia." He was released from the

hospital around Halloween, however a fever, low appetite, irritability, and bruising continued and by Thanksgiving of 1974, he was admitted to Children's Hospital in Pittsburgh. At the time, Timothy had completed only a few months of first grade. "Being that young, I don't remember too much of it." A bone marrow biopsy performed on November 24, 1974, confirmed the diagnosis of acute lymphoblastic leukemia. His symptoms by this time included leg pain, sternal tenderness with fever, anemia, irritability, and bruising.

Timothy's induction therapy started on November 26, 1974 and he left the hospital on December 7, 1974, "And my doctor told my family when they sent me home that I was actually dying." Timothy continued treatment as an outpatient, and until December 24, 1974, he was brought to the hospital every day. The intensified treatment regime began on December 25, 1974, and lasted to February 2, 1975. His treatment regime consisted of the standard chemotherapeutic agents used to combat leukemia: 6-MP, prednisone, intrathecal methotrexate, and vincristine. Timothy was admitted into a central nervous system experimental study and also received prophylactic radiotherapy. He was administered 1800 cGy in 12 treatments to the skull, spinal cord areas, and the genitals. Maintenance therapy began on February 7, 1975, and lasted until November 16, 1979. During these second two phases, visits to the hospital were less frequent. "It went from every day, to once a month, to every couple of months." Timothy's battle with cancer had lasted approximately 5 years.

In January 1980, Timothy had a testicular biopsy performed. It showed immature testicular tissue but no evidence of leukemic cells. He has not had any anticancer therapy since 1979. During his annual checkups now, the doctors do blood work and test his thyroid. "It makes me nervous because [leukemia] is something that you're born with. You can get it back at any time. Although you are cured, it could come back."

TIMOTHY'S REACTIONS TO DIAGNOSIS AND TREATMENT

For 5-year-old Timothy, the hospital stay was a frightening experience. "I remember the first night that [my mom] went home and I was in this big building all by myself. It was a scary thought. I remember I saw visions in the moonlight [on my room wall]." It was also painful.

I remember the first time I had a spinal tap. My parents were supposed be at the hospital but they got stuck in traffic. My mom remembers walking down the hallway and hearing me screaming. They didn't even get to stick the needle in me; they had to wait for my parents to get there.

Timothy was afraid of the needles. "Even when they used to give me blood tests in my fingers, my dad would hold me down and they would try to pry my fingers open. When I get my fingers pricked now, I still jump." He particularly dreaded the monthly bone marrow biopsies. "I dreaded the yellow room because I would go there once a month for the bone marrows. When they put me in the yellow room, I would get real nervous and scared." And his memories of the radiation are still clear. "I remember having red x's on my face. I guess it was actually shooting radiation through me, right in my jaw area." As might be expected, there were complications.

I can remember the first time they took the intravenous off me. They taped a big syringe to my arm so that I could still get intravenous, but now I could go to the playroom and shoot pool or do whatever I wanted to do. Then I became allergic to the tape they wrapped my hand and arm in, and they had to send for a special kind of tape.

The nurses and doctors were kind to Timothy, but not memorable. "I remember some of the nurses but not their names." But he did see the doctors and nurses as a kind of extended family.

The big thing was you couldn't wait to get your school picture taken to take it to their [doctor's office] bulletin board where all their patients would bring their school photos. I would post mine up on the bulletin board. You were like on the "Wall of Fame." They would ask how do you feel in school and are treatments causing you problems in paying attention and learning. You become part of a family. They would watch over you just as your parents would.

To get through the treatments Timothy developed rituals.

I was particular; I was like, everything, was this way. [There was] only one hip that I've ever had my bone marrows in. This finger is the one they always pricked for blood. It's so callused that they can hardly get any blood from it now. I keep telling them it ran out of blood.

He also was "a stubborn little boy . . . a little radical case . . . a troublemaker. Whatever I was told to do, I did the total opposite. And just whatever trouble I could get into, I was in it."

I remember getting a spinal tap once and being told to just lay in bed for the rest of the day. "Don't move. You had a spinal tap." Well, I had to jump out of bed and I hit my spine right where I got a shot. I remember having a headache for 3 days. It was so bad, all I could do [was] lay there with my eyes closed. I couldn't sit up or anything.

Perhaps one of the reasons Timothy treated the hospital treatments so lightly was that he did not know that he was so seriously ill.

All through school I thought I had pneumonia. So, it didn't really affect me knowing that they had given me 3 years to live. I just thought I wasn't feeling too well and I was going through a lot with the treatments.

He didn't even suspect when other children being treated on the same ward didn't make it.

I can still remember one girl in the room next to me; her name was Rachel. They lived in Erie, and they used to come in every day. Her mom and my mom became good friends. But they were treating both of us differently [Rachel was on a different experimental protocol]. It never really hit me that she had the same thing because on the children's ward there were kids that had burns and other things. She felt real sick and she died.

Timothy wasn't told about the leukemia until he was 15.

The day I found out I was driving in the car with my mom. She said, "I have something to tell you. It's very important and it has been on my mind for years." And she looked at me and she started to cry. But she couldn't bring herself to tell me. She said, "There is no Santa Claus." I was like, "Okay, Mom I knew that." So, it was a couple more miles down the road, and she finally brought herself to tell me.

Timothy had several reactions to the news. On the one hand, he felt "like a weight had been lifted off my chest. I actually [knew] what I [had] and I was able to look at it and see what it was all about." On the other hand, "I was scared when my [mom] told me. It astounded me that I could have actually died." Timothy's parents had kept the secret on the advice of the oncologist. "The doctors thought it might be a good idea [for a child of my age] not knowing that you have this disease and you might only have 3 years to live." Timothy seems to agree.

I didn't have that pressure on me of being afraid that I was not going to live any longer. I guess it would be a burden on a young child, knowing that he might not live to be able to play football when he grows up or whatever he wanted to do to plan a life. That's all everyone asks even in school. "What's your goal in life?" Well, if you know that you're not going to make it that long you might just not care about anything and end up depressed. It may make a lot of kids want to give up, as if there is no use trying or fighting to survive. Not knowing helps ease you more than trying to cope and survive. [It helps you] not to be so focused on one thing that might not be worth anything.

When the secret was finally revealed, it seemed to be a great relief to both Timothy's parents and his doctor.

They [Timothy's parents] were worried that I would be mad that they didn't tell me. I wasn't really. Then I couldn't wait to go tell my doctor that my mom finally told me. It seemed to ease him a bit, too. They always used to have me leave the room when he would come in with my blood test results and to talk to my parents.

However, now in retrospect, Timothy can see that not knowing may have caused himself and those around him some embarrassment.

The only problem that came from not knowing was when I would be in health class and we were talking about sickness. I would come up with that I had pneumonia. And everyone would look at me like I was a bit crazy. Then later on finding out it wasn't pneumonia made myself look foolish in class saying that.

Once Timothy found out about the leukemia, he needed to talk to someone.

The day I found out, I had to tell someone. I told my wife. We were just dating at the time. I felt better being able to tell somebody. We were real good friends before we got engaged. She was someone I could talk to. And she just sat and listened and she got a smile on her face. She [said that she] hadn't known it was me. She knew it was one of the kids in my family [but she and her family] thought that it was my younger brother.

TREATMENT SIDE EFFECTS

Timothy's most common complaints throughout the course of his treatment were headaches, vomiting, loss of hair, leg pains, and irritability. He also experienced the bloating associated with taking prednisone. "I was plump . . . heavy. My face was real fat. I remember for the longest time being four feet tall and about four foot round." Once he stopped taking prednisone, he had a difficult time gaining weight. "For the longest time I couldn't get above 75 pounds. Then one day, I finally made it to 76 pounds, and we were like throwing a party."

Most of the side effects eventually disappeared, but a few have persisted.

I still get bad headaches. I can't grow a beard; it won't grow except sometimes in splotches. My teeth are real brittle. Every once in a while, in my right hip [the one used for bone marrow biopsies], I get a burning sensation.

But Timothy is not sterile.

When we [Timothy and his wife] were talking about having kids, I had a doctor's appointment. I asked the doctor if there was a chance I could be sterile. And he said, "With all the radiation and chemotherapy we gave you, there's a strong possibility, a real strong possibility because we gave you extra radiation and chemotherapy." This was on Friday and he told me to call him on Monday [to] set up an appointment [to] get . . . tested. Well, we left my doctor's office and went to my wife's doctor. And then I called him, and I said, "Well, doc, we don't have to take that test; my wife is pregnant." So he said, "I guess we don't have to take that test and congratulations."

IMPACT ON THE FAMILY

When Timothy was initially admitted to Children's Hospital, his mother stayed with him day and night. "They gave her a cot and she could stay in the room." But soon, his mother had to return to work

because they both had to work to help try to pay the bills. It was hard to try and be at work and take care of me, too. My mom would work daylight, and my dad would work at night. When one was going to work, the other was coming home and watching me.

Timothy's father was responsible for transporting him to the hospital, first thing in the morning every day, then eventually less frequently. "I was basically going to the hospital everyday. So, as soon as my dad got home from work, he would drive me straight to Children's Hospital. The ride in [to Pittsburgh from so far away] was the biggest thing." He also tried to ease Timothy's nervousness over the treatments. "My dad would say, 'If it's a good day, maybe you won't have to go to school. We'll go down to Gram's house, so you can eat.' He would try to bribe me, and that would usually work."

Timothy believes "it had to have been a lot of burden for my parents. I put a lot of stress on them." Yet, they gave him strength to get through it.

With my dad and mom there, I always felt I had to be strong, even when I was getting my shots. If I cried, I felt bad because I didn't want to make them worried. I wanted to feel like I was strong, and I was fine with everything going on. It was pride. I didn't want to show my emotions. I wanted to be tough . . . "I can handle it." But meanwhile, down inside, you just wanted to let go . . . to scream.

Timothy "never actually saw my mom crying, but I could hear her crying at nights. Actually both of them would lie in bed and cry. They would wonder what they might have done that God was getting them back." His parents were also very superstitious about what may have caused the leukemia, as they searched for explanations.

I liked roller skating. However, I wasn't allowed to go roller skating because right before I got sick, my mom took me roller skating for the first time. She thought maybe I got [leukemia] from roller skating. Then we got rid of the cat. People told [us] that cats carry leukemia, so they got rid of the cat. It was just anything that she [my mom] thought could have given it to me or anything she heard about at the time because they didn't know a lot about it. Mom and Dad didn't want my brothers to get it. I guess they were being protective so that maybe they wouldn't get it.

Timothy's parents had support from the extended family, and they all conspired to keep the secret of his disease from Timothy. "My whole family kept it from me. My aunts and everybody knew and nobody ever mentioned it." Because of the leukemia, Timothy was probably a little more spoiled by his mother than he might otherwise have been. "No matter where we went shopping, if I said I wanted something, I got what I wanted and my younger brother would, too. They just couldn't buy for me; they had to buy for him, too." But his father worked hard to make him toe the line.

When I went out for football, I had a coach who would say, "Don't hit him too hard" or "You only have to run two laps instead of five laps." But then my dad became the football coach and it wasn't like that with my dad. If he had the rest of the team running five laps, then you ran five laps. You know, I wasn't treated special. If I was doing something wrong, he pulled me off the field and put me on the bench just as quick as he would anybody else out there.

Still, his parents tried to protect him as much as they could from it and it showed in subtle ways.

My parents never got my second-grade picture because of the fact they didn't want me seeing a picture and being upset that I am the kid in the picture, and I don't have hair. So out of all my school pictures, the second-grade [picture] is the only one missing.

THE SCHOOL EXPERIENCE

During the initial stages of his illness, Timothy "received no education or instruction." Yet he remembers that "while I was at the hospital, for a couple of weeks, my parents were bringing me my schoolwork from school. Then my parents would go over it with me, and I would do it." Strange as it may seem (being so ill), Timothy was grateful for the diversion. "It would actually give me something to do at the hospital, other than just laying there wondering what is going on or something." After a few months, when his parents realized that Timothy would not be returning to school for some time, they arranged for a tutor. "That helped me pass first grade and be able to go on to second grade. I wasn't actually in school because of all the treatments and radiation . . . I couldn't go to school." The tutoring became a routine part of Timothy's life.

The tutor came to the house Monday though Friday from noon to 4 o'clock. She would go over reading, math, spelling, or whatever. She was very much aware of my illness. My parents had told her what was going on and everything. They told her if she had any questions to call the doctors and they would give her information. I am not sure if she ever did that.

Timothy was not an eager student.

I remember she made me sit there and learn. I was a little kid and I didn't want to sit there; I wanted to watch TV or something since I was home. But she also made it fun to learn. She taught me by making a game out of something to try and learn. She was very persistent with me, but also made it fun. It wasn't like she was the old schoolteacher with a ruler, smacking your fingers or whatever. We would sit at the kitchen table and she would give me a notebook to write down my spelling words. If I did well, she would give me a star on a chart. If I got x amount of stars on a chart within that week or whatever, she would give me something special or let me have an extra treat for the day. This would give me the ambition to do the work. I was learning schoolwork but I was having fun doing it. She would leave me homework but I knew the next day I would be rewarded for it.

Despite the fact that Timothy had a tutor, his first-grade teacher stayed in close contact with the family.

My first-grade teacher would always come up to visit me and drop off work for me. She would show me what to do for a couple of pages. I would try to understand what to do and she would ask if I had any questions. She'd stay until I would get started on math or English to make sure I understood what to do. Then she would leave and I would finish it on my own.

She also tried to keep Timothy in touch with his first-grade classmates.

She would have the kids sign cards for me and maybe in art class they would make something for me. This helped me [to know] that I still had friends and they were thinking about me. It was easier for the kids when I went back to school because they knew I had been sick and that they were not going to get sick because I was sick.

Still, returning to second grade was not easy for Timothy.

It was difficult leaving home to go back to school because you felt you were learning at home. Why go back? Why can't I stay at home? I was nervous going back to school. You know, because they haven't seen you for almost a year. I was wondering how they were going to accept me bald and swollen. I thought if I got too close to someone, they would back up away from me like, "Don't come near me. Don't touch me."

His parents thought he should wear a wig.

I was almost completely bald. My parents had me fitted for a wig. They had it cut the same way as my hair was. [But] I didn't want it on. They [explained to me that] no one will know. I can remember them telling me a couple of people in our family that were guys wore wigs. One of my cousins was in security and he wore a wig to work. [But] it was the fact that I knew and so as long as I had the feeling that I knew I had it on, I felt that everybody else knew that I had it on. If I would have been forced to wear it, I think I would have been a lot more uncomfortable in school, thinking that people were maybe joking about me if I had seen anyone looking at me or pointing toward me. I would have been real nervous.

So instead, Timothy kept his head covered with a sailor's cap.

Just being myself made me feel a lot better. I was I. I wasn't someone under a wig. I wasn't going to be made up to be what they wanted to see. I was able to be myself and it helped everyone to accept me. I still feel that way today. If you can't accept me for what I am, then forget about you. You're not worth bothering with.

Wearing the cap broke school rules. "The rule was no one was allowed to wear caps in school . . . students or faculty. But they let me wear a sailor's cap." It also produced a nickname that followed him through school. "They all ended up calling me 'Popeye' in school. So, my doctor heard about this and when I would go in for my shot every Friday, he would call it Popeye juice. Popeye had his spinach and I was getting my juice. It helped me a lot because I was nervous [about getting shots]."

Timothy's parents valued education and were involved in helping him keep up with his schoolwork.

My parents set rules for me to do my homework. They went over a lot with me especially when I was in the hospital. Even when I went back to school, you did your homework before you played and they would check it. And if something was wrong, my dad would make a mark and then he would leave it up to me to figure out what was wrong instead of just [saying], "Here is the answer." This is the way it was done. He would make me sit there and figure it out. If I got to a point that I was really stuck, then he would sit there and work it out with me until I got the answer and understood it. He used to say, "You've got to understand how to do it before you can do it."

They also tried hard to keep educational concerns in the foreground.

They still viewed education as important even though I was battling leukemia. I think it helped them to not give up on me. They never told me, "You're only going to live this long so don't bother with it." They didn't give up hope and think, "Why worry about it because it is not going to matter in his life anyway?" My parents were a major contribution in helping me get through [school].

It was Timothy's parents who took on the responsibility for contacting the school and keeping them informed about his treatments and progress. The medical personnel had no contact with the school even though Timothy went through 2 more years of treatment after returning to school.

The teachers were more or less informed by my parents . . . finding out what was going on. Then the teachers would inform each other. It wasn't the medical personnel; it was my parents.

When Timothy was ready to return to school at the beginning of second grade

I think my mom just told them I was coming back and that I might be a little behind the other kids in what they learned since I was going through a tutor, and not being taught daily with them.

She also told them that "they might have to spend extra time with me to get me caught up" and the teachers seemed quite willing to do that. "The teachers helped because they knew you were behind and took the extra time with you."

Timothy often missed school because of his treatments.

Depending on how I felt after the treatment determined whether I went back to school or not. I did miss a good bit of school because there were times you could just not be feeling great, and all of a sudden your stomach would get queasy and sick . . . and nausea . . . and

everything. It was pretty legitimate. Mainly, the only times I stayed at home was [on days when I had] my doctor's appointments, on Fridays.

His teachers were very cooperative about helping him make up missed work.

Sometimes, I would just miss the morning and the teacher would give me what I missed for homework. Occasionally, I would stay after school for a half hour or so and the teacher would go over what I had missed and help me out. It was hard always trying to catch up with the other kids.

And he seldom abused his right to stay at home if he was sick.

I do remember one time, I faked my temperature. My mom walked out of the room, and my cup of tea was sitting right there. Well, I just stuck [the thermometer] in my cup of tea. It broke the thermometer. So my mom said, "I know you did something because the thermometer broke and your temperature isn't that high."

Another way that Timothy's teachers helped him keep up with his schoolwork was to provide him with a peer-partner.

The teachers would sometimes have kids pair up with me in the room. They would help me. If we were like starting multiplication or division or something, they would pair me up with a smarter kid in the class to try to help me . . . while they were teaching everybody else . . . this person kept me caught up. I could ask them questions instead of sitting there totally lost in class and having to say I don't know what's going on and the teacher would then have to stop the class. I was teamed up with students a lot.

This partnering made Timothy feel important "because I was getting to work with someone else and no one else was. I suppose I was actually being treated different but it made you feel good about yourself." Humor also kept Timothy on an even keel.

I learned how to make jokes about [the illness and its consequences] and it helped put everyone at ease. You know, if I started laughing about it, then it was okay for them to start laughing. I remember doing somersaults in sym, and when I did a somersault, there was a pile of hair lying there on the mat. I tried to make it a joke to help ease it a bit from what I recall. They weren't laughing or joking or making fun of me because I guess they really didn't understand.

Throughout elementary school, there were no counseling services available to Timothy, but he felt well taken care of. "There were some older students that took me under their wing. If anyone said anything to me and they heard it . . . they would let that person know about it." Of course, "once in a while in the older grades someone might point at you and giggle, but no one ever really confronted me." Timothy also stayed in close contact with his first-grade tutor. "I actually looked forward to her coming because I had someone sit there with me and we would talk. When I started back to school, she would still stop by sometimes because [school] was so upsetting to me." And once back at school, he found he could engage some of the teachers in needed conversations.

Sometimes, after school I'd stay behind to do the erasers and walk home from school so that the teacher would sit and talk to me. There was no school psychologist. It's hard to talk about it. I really didn't know how to tell people about the pain. It was never brought up. I kept a lot in me . . . I kept a lot inside.

In fact, Timothy thought his "teachers were great and they were always telling me to take it easy or they would watch me on the playground." By junior high, Timothy found he could talk with the dean.

I never attended a special class. The only special services I received were in junior high and senior high, you had a dean you could talk to. In elementary school, there wasn't anyone really to talk to. I never really talked to too many people about it because I didn't find out what it was until I was 15.

And Timothy never felt left out or isolated, even when he first returned to school after being out for a year.

It being a small town and everybody knowing each other might have helped them in accepting me. Most of the kids saw me during the summertime. Some were probably stunned. I think if I would have gone back to school at the junior high level, I probably would have been harassed more. I think being young had a lot to do with me being accepted back into the school.

Timothy made regular progress through school. He was always considered an average student and he was never retained. That, Timothy thought, was very important.

It made you feel good about yourself that okay I passed and I am going on to the next grade. It wasn't like oh man, I've got to go through this all again. Your friends are going on to the next grade and you're not . . . so they taunt you . . . because then you are considered dumb, not being smart enough. Then you sit back and think it might be because of your illness or maybe I am dumb. You shouldn't use your illness as an excuse.

Because of his illness and treatments, Timothy's parents were in constant communication with the school.

The school would call my parents if they thought I looked like I was getting sick. And my parents anytime something was wrong or if they thought I was hurting . . . they would call the school to see how I was doing and making sure everything was okay. I was home for a whole year and then all of a sudden, I'm not there anymore during the day. They just wanted to make sure I was fine.

Timothy's parents also became quite active in school activities, so that they would be around to take care of him. "My mom joined the PTA and helped with class parties and my dad became involved with the Cub Scouts and became the football coach. They became more involved than they probably would have otherwise."

Although during most of his schooling, Timothy did not know what was the matter with him, he assumes that his teachers knew and "just seemed to accept it. I guess being in school they had just known what was going on and they were just trying to make it a lot easier." Once he was told about the leukemia, "I started reading about it and got into it and what it was about. It really scared me. But then I realized that the treatments really did help me."

I remember in high school, I needed to pass health to graduate. So what I did was I finally sat down and did a report on leukemia . . . what it was about and all the treatments and everything. At the end of the report, I said I really believe the treatments do work. My teacher, in front of the class, said, "Well, why do you believe that?" And I said, "Because I survived. It worked for me." There were kids in the class with tears in their eyes. And the teacher marked down an "A". I passed the class.

AREAS OF SCHOOL DIFFICULTY

During the 2 years that he was receiving treatments while going to school, Timothy was very distracted. After he had been told about the leukemia, the treatments weighed heavily on his mind, and that caused him to daydream and lose information or fall behind in class.

When I was being tutored, it was one on one. So, you were prone to sit there and pay attention. But once I was back in school and thinking, there would be times in class that I would just start daydreaming about the treatments that I was having. . . . You know, I would think that in a couple of days I have to go to the doctors or have to have a bone marrow on Friday. . . . So, you'd think about all these things and the next thing you know the bell rings and the class is over and you're like what did we just do in class today. Especially once I found out what had happened to me, it had me thinking a lot more than before.

Timothy also experienced comprehension and memory problems (focus of attention), for both oral and written material.

I have a hard time memorizing stuff. I have to go over it and over it. It's short term. Sometimes in the middle of a conversation, when the person is still talking, I realize that I don't understand. I didn't hear a word they said. Also, I [would] read something and go through it, and then, it's like what did I read? And I [would] read it again. Maybe I have to read it a couple of times to comprehend it. It is like I read something but I don't know what it is trying to tell me. And I read it again. I misinterpreted on how something was phrased or I took a word a wrong way or something like that. I would read something and then say to myself, well what did I actually read?

Often, Timothy was "totally lost" in class, but he felt uncomfortable about asking for help.

You don't want special treatment but yet you do want to be able to say if you're having problems, to feel comfortable to ask questions . . . but in school I didn't. I found myself sitting back a lot. Instead of asking questions and being nervous, you just go on your own. Instead of saying I don't understand, I guess I just faked it and I was totally lost.

There were areas of school in which Timothy did fairly well, such as writing, spelling, and mathematics. In the remodeling business with his dad, he uses a lot of math, and he reports no problems with it.

SURVIVING

Timothy's outlook on the entire ordeal is basically positive and he is happy to share his success with others.

When I am at the doctor's office for an annual checkup for something, the doctor might ask me to talk to a little boy there. The doctor tells the parents that I had leukemia and that I might not have made it. I go right in and talk to him and tell him, "I played football. I played baseball. You can do that, too. Don't let it hold you back. Go for whatever you want to go for. You can still do it." While I talk, you can see the parents easing a bit . . . that maybe their child will one day be able to do normal things again. It was like an honor to be able to talk about it. If I could help one person, it makes me feel better.

But the experience itself was not always positive.

It doesn't make you an outcast because you have it. It makes you feel like an outcast because of the side effects, like losing your hair or swelling. It makes you feel like you're not the same as everybody else.

And Timothy often wants to just put the experience behind him. "It's something in the past. I mean, some people are leery to talk about it. If it's mentioned, you can see people getting nervous." Still, it is always with him.

I make sure I still go to my appointments and they will tell me to watch this or that for my health. Don't wear yourself out. Don't drain yourself. Make sure you get x amount of hours sleep. Eat healthy.

And it was a particular worry when his wife was pregnant.

I was always thinking what kind of effect would it have on the baby. You know . . . is it going to have 10 fingers and 10 toes? Is it going to be healthy? Is anything I went through going to jeopardize the baby in any way? And it didn't. I have two healthy kids and I hope they stay that way.

Despite the worrying, Timothy smokes cigarettes. He had started smoking when he was about 14 or 15, before he "found out I had leukemia." He understands the dangers of smoking but he can't seem to quit. He smokes "a half a pack a day."

I wish I could stop because I know smoking causes cancer and I already beat it once. But I am just a cranky person if I don't smoke. Once in a while, my daughter who is 4, she sees me with cigarettes and she'll go "nah, nah, nah." I know my chances are greater because I already had cancer. I would like to quit. If it comes to the point where someone told me either you quit smoking or you're going to have to go through those treatments all over again . . . that would probably finally make me do it cold turkey. I would quit because of the treatments. There was a lot of pain involved in it. And being older, I think it would be more painful because my bones aren't as soft as they were when I was younger. And going through the bone marrows and spinal taps . . . I don't think I'd be able to deal with that pain as much I did when I was younger.

Except for the smoking, finding out about cancer changed Timothy's perspective about day-to-day living.

I became more cautious and more aware of what I am doing. I figure I got a second chance at life. And most people don't get that. So, I try to take full advantage of whatever I am able to do . . . like even being with my kids. When I found out I had leukemia, it made you stop and think . . . not to take advantage . . . be happy . . . and accept things for what they are.

It also changed and affected his relationships. "Of course, there is a greater attachment to my parents because of what we went through and survived." And it has affected his marriage.

Once in a while, it might cause a problem. My wife makes a remark like, "You are Mommy and Daddy's boy." Then she ends up regretting it. But it bothers her because she feels that she hurt me by saying something like that. Actually, it doesn't really affect me her saying something like that.

And like other cancer survivors, Timothy has tried to find some meaning in his triumph over disease.

Every day I thank God upstairs that He left me here for a reason. I've had a second chance. That's the positive effect of it all. It makes you enjoy things more instead of taking everything for granted. One guy told me never to play the lottery. He says, "You've already won." Not everybody gets a second chance at life. He said to me, "You've had it. You've had your lottery." My lottery is more than money; it is life itself. I've actually won the lottery, and it's life.

6

What Makes the Difference?

Matthew's Story

What really makes the difference in the way we experience
life is what we believe about ourselves and what we
believe is possible for ourselves.

—John Marks Templeton

Matthew is 27 years old, the youngest of four children with one brother
and two sisters. He works as a blacksmith and lives in a medium-sized
town east of Pittsburgh. He is slender in build, about 5'7", with sandy-
colored hair and mustache. He is single. His reaction to the interview was
candid. "I always thought that probably some day I would hear from
somebody. I always did expect it. And maybe this is it." Yet conflicts about
disclosure permeated the interview. "I always thought I would never want
to talk about it. But I am really here sitting talking to you."

Matthew views himself as a positive, happy-go-lucky, optimistic person. He appeared pleased to be able to tell what he knew about his illness and to contribute to helping others who may be facing what he had
had to handle. Due to his memory difficulties acquired from the treatments, he was often slow in recounting the events, but in his struggle to
do so, he was able to express an interesting and informative description
of his experience.

ONSET OF THE DISEASE AND TREATMENT

In September 1973, Matthew was in a wedding and had his picture taken at that event. Approximately, 1 month later, in October, Matthew had his picture taken at school. Distinctive changes between these two pictures alerted first his grandmother and subsequently his mother that something was wrong. In the second photo, Matthew was extremely pale and his hair was turning much lighter. By December, his mother finally took him to the family doctor.

Our family doctor noticed that I was awfully pale. For some reason he drew blood, and got hold of Children's Hospital. Maybe if it wasn't for him it would have been too late, but he caught it. I owe him a lot.

The family doctor sent them directly to the local hospital for more blood tests. Matthew was confined to his bed to prevent bruising and was given iron to combat his anemia. By the January 24, 1974, Matthew was admitted to Children's Hospital of Pittsburgh with swelling of the cervical (neck and back), axillary, and inguinal (groin) nodes. On January 25, a bone marrow biopsy was performed and Matthew was diagnosed, at the age of 7, with acute lymphoblastic leukemia. "I remember staying [at the hospital]. I assumed that they kept me right away as soon as they realized what it was."

Matthew was admitted to an experimental protocol on January 27.

I remember when they [doctors] were going to put us all in three [experimental] groups which you didn't know what group you were going to be put in to. It was described to me that some had all the treatment, some had half the treatment, and some had no treatment. And that was the only way that they could find what was helping you. I was in the full treatment group.

His initial hospital stay was 12 days. He was administered prednisone, vincristine, and L-asparaginase until March 3, 1974.

Over the next 3 weeks, he received 2,400 cGy of radiation in 18 treatments to the central nervous system, 1,250 cGy to the thymus, and 1,200 cGy to the kidneys, liver, spleen, and testicles. At the same time, he began an intensive regime of 6-MP and intrathecal methotrexate.

I remember getting radiation to my head and lying underneath it and a light coming on with crosshairs on it. I got that on the head, neck, chest, and genitals. The second study group might have only had it in the chest and genitals and not the head. So, it just depended on what group you were in. I got it everywhere.

Matthew went into maintenance chemotherapy on April 11, 1974; this phase of treatment lasted until March 25, 1979.

It was a lot. You were scared. It just seemed like you never got any rest even when you came home. If you had a week at home, it wasn't like you could get back into it because it seemed like you had to go again. But then it all became routine. It just became what you did. That's what you had to do to be here.

His entire chemotherapy regime lasted approximately 5 years.

After all therapy had ended, Matthew had a testicular biopsy that showed atrophy of the testes but no leukemic infiltrates. "They also checked the bone marrow pretty often through the years. I used to hate that . . . [it was] really painful." Matthew has received no anticancer therapy since March 1979.

I still go in once a year . . . as long as everything keeps looking good. I was surprised to hear that some people don't. They just disappear. Maybe they are afraid of what they'll hear. Once you've had it [cancer], you think, "what's keeping it from coming back again?" Does lightning strike a place twice? I believe it can and it does.

MATTHEW'S REACTIONS TO THE DIAGNOSIS AND TREATMENT

In the beginning, Matthew did not understand why he was so sick. "It was the beginning of first grade. I never really fathomed what was going on." But he knew it was serious. "You can pick it up from your parents that it was something serious." And although they did not tell him what was wrong with him, his parents did invite him to help make decisions about treatment.

I remember my mom asked if I wanted to go through with it. It was going to be a lot, and it was going to be long, and I didn't have to. I mean, you were 7 years old. And I really didn't think, "Well, yea, why not?" I remember saying distinctly, "Yea, if it's what you want and it will help." I remember saying it.

Matthew remembers that "everyone [at the hospital] was really, really nice. Everybody was cooperative. They made you feel you were the only one being treated . . . like you were the only one in the hospital." The doctors made him feel important. "The doctor [in charge of the experimental protocol] always said you were a pioneer. And the nurses were kind. "I remember one of the [nurses] used to stop in every night and make sure I didn't want anything before I went to bed."

But he feels some conflict over the fact that he was selected for the full treatment group. On the one hand, he can say,

Nobody survived with the no treatment. Even with the half treatment, most of them didn't [make it]. It just depended on when it was caught and how your body reacted to [the treatment]. I'm thankful that I was put in the right group. I mean you had to be thankful that they had some kind of treatment.

On the other hand, he believes in his heart, "I would have probably survived with the half treatment and half the side effects."

TREATMENT SIDE EFFECTS

Matthew experienced the usual array of transient side effects.

I remember not having any hair. I wore a Pittsburgh Pirate ball cap. I remember being plump [from the prednisone]. My face was round and I was never like that before. I was very nauseated all the time. You always felt that food tasted like wax. My mother and grandmother would yell at me to eat. But if it tastes like wax, you don't want to eat.

He also experienced some long-term side effects from the treatment regime. He had difficulty growing a beard. "I probably didn't even get to grow a moustache until I was 21 years old. Also, my hair is really thin." And Matthew is shorter than his father and his siblings. "My oldest sister is six foot. My brother is six foot. My dad's height is close to five foot ten. My height is about five foot seven. They said I would have probably been two or three inches taller." Neither of these long-term side effects concern Matthew. "I guess it's no big deal."

But Matthew is concerned about the fact that he is probably sterile. "I've never got tested because the doctor said he was 99.9% sure I was sterile. He said I could get tested but he also said anyone that got the radiation in that area is going to be sterile." His concern has been heightened by his recent engagement. You have to discuss that when you get into a relationship.

I've had a few different girlfriends that I've never said anything to because in the back of your mind it wasn't that serious. So, you let it ride. I have a girlfriend now and she's going through a divorce. She has two kids. I sometimes think well . . . yea . . . because I can't have them, so there they are.

Matthew has tried to be philosophical about it.

They didn't tell me until I was probably dating age. I think they told my mom and dad. It took my mom and dad a lot to tell me. No big deal. I'm here. I mean that's secondary to what [could have happened]. Maybe that would bother some people, but I was thinking, "no, that's secondary."

Still, there is obvious apprehension and reservations.

Maybe it was supposed to be. If there was a pregnancy, I'd have to be afraid . . . I'd feel sick to my stomach over it . . . if I were to have a baby. I thought about that for years. That would scare the heck out of me. It would worry me that [something would be wrong with the baby].

IMPACT ON THE FAMILY

Matthew's parents were very supportive throughout the ordeal. "I re-member [my parents] staying until they couldn't stay any longer. It had to have worn them out. [Then,] I remember my mom and dad coming up every day. Once he was released from the hospital, "my father was the one who worked and my mother stayed home and took care of me. She had to make sure I took my medication."

Matthew and his parents suspected that his leukemia was the result of their living close to the nuclear power plant [when Matthew was young].

We always wondered if it had anything to do with [the nuclear power plant] because we didn't live too far from that. And there were a few kids right within the same area [who developed leukemia, too]. I remember distinctly as a kid riding a pony. And this was before I was diagnosed. And I remember sitting on that pony. Then a few months later, I was diagnosed with this. I remember my parents saying the pony had died and there wasn't anything wrong with the pony. There were a few cows in that pasture that died, too. Maybe whatever settled on their backs I absorbed from riding the pony. Also, all the other kids that were in that area who got sick [had leukemia] too were east of that power plant. Perhaps the wind blew in that direction.

Matthew's parents told very few people that he had cancer.

Nobody knew except our immediate family and close family friends. My grandparents, some aunts and uncles, and maybe a close friend to my mom and dad. A few people like that. I have a brother and two sisters. They are all older. They all knew. But they all must have kept it pretty hush-hush.

They also did not talk to him about it very much. "Whenever you were of age to understand the whole concept . . . the whole deal, it was up to you to tell . . . talk about it . . . or not to talk about it." Matthew believes that this was a good decision on their part. "I just am really grateful that they left me do what I wanted and needed to do and [gave] me the chance to decide when it was time [to talk about it]."

Because they insisted on keeping the illness private, there were no fund-raisers to help cover medical expenses.

I remember money was hard especially because they kept it under their hat. I mean, even today, you go into a 7-Eleven to get gas, and there might be a little milk carton there, and it will say a fund for whoever . . . a situation just like mine. And I always drop a little bit of money in it.

Again, Matthew believes that this was the right choice.

I was grateful to my parents, to this day, that they didn't do that to me. They gave me a chance just to be me. And nobody had to know anything. It would have helped them financially. But I give them credit that they gave me a chance to just be like everybody else. Maybe [having fund-raisers] would have never affected anything but then maybe it would have.

The trade-off was that Matthew's parents managed to provide him with a very calm and secure environment.

Everything was pretty calm. It made it nice for me. It was a steady, calm, and secure environment. My dad must have guessed . . . put himself in my place or something. It was a gift. He figured that's how he would have wanted it, so he chose that for me.

And, Matthew believes that by not telling people about his illness, he was given the opportunity to become someone other than "a boy who is different, a boy with cancer." "When I was growing up, you didn't want anybody to know you were different. Not that you were . . . but you kind of felt you were. It would have been hard to grow up with explaining it all the time."

When Matthew talked about his parents, it was with tender affection, admiration, and respect.

I feel I had a great raising. They let you become who you were to be but yet they were shoving you in a direction that I should be going in. I remember [my parents] saying, "Are you happy that's the way we did it?" And I said to them, "Elated."

They modeled a matter-of-fact way of handling adversity, and it helped him get through the illness and the treatments.

Sometimes I heard my parents get upset but then it was just something God handed down, and you just dealt with it. I was always raised that way. Whatever happened, happened, and you just dealt with the situation. You don't want to die. So . . . you just did it.

THE SCHOOL EXPERIENCE

Matthew attended a Catholic school from first grade to graduation. During the first month or two of first grade, prior to his diagnosis, Matthew didn't go out to play on the playground with the other children, but stood by the window of the classroom instead. Also, Matthew cut the front of his hair off using school scissors, one day. Matthew never came right out and said he was feeling sick or was having pain—he must have had a very high tolerance for pain—but the doctors believe that these behaviors were nonverbal outcries to the adults around Matthew to grab their attention and clue them into the fact that something was wrong. However, the nun who was his teacher never notified Matthew's parents.

Matthew was out of school from January of first grade through to the end of the school year; once he was home from the hospital, a tutor was assigned to him.

When I came home from the hospital and it was known that I would be out the rest of first grade, a nun from first grade was admitted into my parents' confidence and came to the house to tutor me. She treated me like a little angel. I remember wearing my hat and being tutored. You did things just like school. Paperwork. If you didn't do this, then when you went back to school, you weren't in the same place as the others.

Matthew returned to school in second grade. "When I went back to school, I was mostly just trying to get past those first few days of being nervous. Then once you passed that, it was no big deal." Matthew is certain that the combination of being in a Catholic school environment and having nuns as teachers contributed to his having a successful and positive reintegration into school.

I don't know how the teachers dealt with it. I would assume the teachers had to have known because I was wearing a ball cap at school. I just had a feeling they knew and they looked out for me without saying anything . . . like a guardian angel . . . out there watching me. Like I said, maybe I had an edge going to a Catholic school. Instead of having 30 or 40 kids in a class [in a public school], the Catholic schools would have only 18 or 20 in a class. I have to believe that had a lot to do with it.

Nobody made a fuss over Matthew, and he wasn't singled out for special treatment.

I think maybe I got slightly spoiled. I wasn't really disciplined a lot. If you were bad [in school], you got the ruler across your knuckles. I was good but I do remember getting the ruler across my knuckles once or twice.

And he always felt well taken care of.

I always felt the teachers kind of looked out for you. They never made you feel like you were the odd one out. They just looked out enough that if a kid asked a question and the teacher heard it, she caught it some way. And in that way they made you feel comfortable returning [to school].

Matthew believes "it must have been hard for the teachers" but that they helped make things go very smoothly.

When I went back to school [in second grade], I still had to go once or twice a week for treatments. I was nauseated in school [but] I don't remember any gut-wrenching explanations I had to make or anything. So, it must have been all right. It just worked out.

He also believes that "the kids picked up on that attitude [of the teachers]" and that they, too, "just left it ride."

It might have been a lot rougher. I suppose if they had noticed when I was in school that I wore a hat because I had no hair and I was lousy in gym class, and then you couldn't read, well, then maybe it would have been a bigger thing because the kids would have put it together and said some things. So, if you were lucky enough only to have one of those things wrong with you like no hair, then everything was all right.

Matthew doesn't remember any negative reactions from the students.

When I first came home from the hospital, three little boys stopped at the house unannounced. They asked my mother what happened to my hair. My mother simply told them it was from the medicine, and that seemed to be enough of an explanation. They stayed and played with me and never said anything about it again.

One explanation he offered for acceptance on the part of the other students was that "we were all young. You could tell kids anything then and they went along with you." Or, "maybe it was that you stayed with the same group of kids from first grade to eighth grade. Once they understood, they always understood, so we never had to explain it anymore to the whole class." But, in fact, Matthew believes that no one ever explained it to his classmates even once.

They [the teachers] never said, "Oh look. Little Matthew's back and he's been gone for so long. Isn't everyone happy to see him?" And if they did, they must have done it before I came back, which I can't imagine that either because what would you have told the kids? They would still have too many questions. So, they must have never said anything. As far as anyone knew, nobody was different.

And none of his classmates ever said anything to him about his illness or his appearance. "No one made fun of my hair or ball cap. No one asked how come I got to wear it."

I have one kid I am still in touch with today. He was in school with me in first grade. He knew something was wrong. But he never asked and never treated me different . . . never did anything. I just ran into him again a few years ago. And he said, "Is everything all right? I never did ask in all those years, so, is everything all right, huh?" And I said, "Yea, I'm here."

Matthew believes that not telling anyone, and not talking about the cancer or the treatment, were the right courses of action for him. "When you're growing up, kids can be really cruel and they might have picked on you about your hair loss or something." But Matthew isn't certain a family could get away with that course of action today.

You know I can't imagine kids [with leukemia] going [back to school] now and no one saying anything, because . . . of the way kids are today. I mean, one of my girlfriend's children is a little girl. She's in the third grade and boy, is she smart as a top. So, if you were diagnosed that late, at age 8 or 9, maybe it would be a lot different because kids are smarter and they have a lot more questions and are more curious. Because, boy, you wouldn't get anything past her.

AREAS OF SCHOOL DIFFICULTY

Matthew openly admitted to difficulties in school during and after his treatment for ALL.

I was never an A student. I was lousy in spelling and math. I remember in school you always had to learn 10 to 20 words. I would remember them that night. I just memorized the word and pictured it. So, when I went in the next day to do the test, you just wrote them down and you passed. But, after that, I didn't remember how to spell the words. So, I can't spell anything. Like if I had to sit down and write you a paragraph, it would be distinctive. I would have to use a dictionary. As for my handwriting, I never learned how to flow. They always said I drew my letters and never learned how to let them flow.

Matthew also has difficulty with long-term and short-term memory.

I can remember things about history or something that happened in first grade but I can't remember I have an appointment or whatever. If it's like, "Grab me a pack of cigarettes on your way home," it just goes in here and out here [pointing to his ears]. [In school], as I studied it I would remember it for the next day. It's like taking a picture of it and you could see it. So, whenever it was time to do the test, I would remember it. I could pass the test that week, but the following week, if I was given the same test, I wouldn't pass. But if someone just mentioned something to me, then I don't remember what was said. I can remember some things from a long time ago but I can't remember from two months ago. And I can't remember people's names for nothing.

Matthew feels that these memory problems were related to having been in the full treatment experimental group. "I mentioned it to the doctor the last time I talked to him. He said he had given me radiation to the brain. So there's a strong possibility."

But the learning problems did not make school a stressful experience for Matthew. His parents "really didn't push me about school" and Matthew "never played on it. They say your mind is 10 times more powerful than you'll ever use. So maybe my own subconscious got me through it." Matthew was glad that no one ever suggested that he get special help in school.

I wouldn't have gone for special help because then somebody would know [about the leukemia]. So, you just always wanted to slip back in when you had to come back [to school]. It just worked out for me. I'm glad it was maybe just luck.

All in all, Matthew has fond memories of school and of the teachers who taught him.

I remember a few of the sisters were older and I remember one in particular . . . she used to always ask if I was all right but she would never do it in front of people. If it was like open house and my parents were late, then I remember her asking. She wasn't a "nebby" lady. And she would always pat me. I remember she would always rub me on the head or pat me on the back. And she would always say, "I'm always praying for you." I remember, I had to stop in [the elementary] school for something when I was in high school and so I went down to see her. And she said, "I'm still praying for you today. . . . every day, you know. I can't forget." In the back of your mind, you remember that little sister. It's just really weird that this woman would think of me every day.

SURVIVING

Survival from anything traumatic leaves a residue of memories and feelings. Surviving often requires some soul searching and working through the debris of what has happened. Matthew struggled throughout his young life to not become a cancer survivor, to not have the illness "mold his life."

I just didn't want to be molded. I didn't want other people to push me in a direction and make a big issue out of [my having leukemia]. When you're a little kid, when you're 7 years old, you are trying to be accepted. Usually no matter how bad you want to be who you are the pressure is too, too strong to be who everybody else is. I didn't ever want to be forced to be not who you really are. I don't know if everybody's had that chance or wanted it. Maybe that little girl I mentioned that had the fund-raising thing . . . maybe that's how she wanted it. Maybe that made her feel comfortable that everybody knew, that you had this big crowd behind you . . . rooting you on. For me, it was inside. It came from within. I just walked to my own beat. I was my own drummer. And I am grateful that I had that chance. If I didn't, I would have been formed by other people.

Now, Matthew is also struggling to not "become his career."

I went to community college for 2 years for criminal justice. I didn't finish, though. I wasn't really interested in it. Everything that you go to college for is for a career not a job, and I never wanted a career . . . because that is something you become. You become your career. So, if you're a doctor, then you become that doctor. I started out to become a state policeman [but] even then that's what you become. I always thought I'd rather be like my dad. He had a job . . . you come home and that's it. Who you are is who you are. I was interested in shoeing. I'm a blacksmith. Everyone thinks it is a dying trade but there are a lot of people who do it and there are a lot of horses.

One of the most difficult issues for Matthew remains his conflict over disclosure. All his life, he, his parents, and his doctors have stressed the importance of not disclosing his survivor status.

I remember once splitting my head open. I was 14 years old or . . . maybe a little older. The neighbor took me to the hospital. I used the local hospital. I couldn't get anyone to treat me because I needed a consent. There wasn't anybody home right at the time. Finally my sister came home and they got in touch with her. They asked if there was anything they should know for treatment. It was just some stitches in my head and send you home. But she was only a few years older than me, in her early 20s, and she was scared. So she said I had leukemia. Boy, then they wanted to know all kinds of stuff. They wanted to know it all and they pumped her for information. I remember my mom and dad got really mad at my sister. Now, they wouldn't quit wanting to know. You have to be careful with jobs and insurances. No matter what I do in my life, they want to know your background . . . diseases or anything. I always write no. I think that is why my mom was so upset because my sister had mentioned it to [the hospital]. They recorded it.

The doctors had reassured Matthew that his hospital records were confidential and that "there's no way that they could ever find out. He was the only who would ever know." And Matthew has been very deliberate about not letting people know.

If by some small chance, something comes up and somebody is talking about it . . . you just really don't say anything. I think that's why I never studied about it. You know all this information. Then, somebody would say, "Boy, did you have it or did you have to write a book about it?" So, you didn't study it.

He didn't want people to have expectations about what he should do or be.

You never know how people are going to react to that. They make it really hard for you. When everybody knows [you had cancer], they have a question in their minds or watch what you do in your life. I don't have to do anything, or I can do whatever. And maybe when it's all done, I can make it in privacy. That's what it is all about for me.

Matthew has worked hard to "just lead a normal life."

Leukemia is pretty big and a lot of people don't survive, but it is not like your nose is going to be upside down for the rest of your life and you have to deal with it. It's like once you're out of the water, you're as normal as anybody else is.

But more recently, he has come to realize that keeping the secret

doesn't matter anymore. I always thought one day when I become somebody then I would say I had this [leukemia]. [Now] I know I made a Matthew . . . at least according to myself in life. There are always a million things that you want to do. I've done enough things . . . past the point that most people don't do. Now, if anybody would find out, for instance, it wouldn't matter to me . . . and it wouldn't affect or change who I am because I am already who I am going to be. So, right now it doesn't matter and I don't care who knows.

Matthew does not dwell on the impact that surviving leukemia has had on his life. "Some people might have made a really big deal out of it where it really made an impact on their lives. And others just dealt with it." Still, he recognizes that "I am a stronger and more sensitive person on the inside [because of surviving leukemia]." And he is ready "to help [others] if I could in any way.

My doctor said that [I] could show people and kids growing up that they could have a normal life. This [going through leukemia] is just a short time in their lives but they will be all right. It's not like never ending.

At the same time, it all happened so long ago.

I was just thinking about it not too long ago about getting a book and reading more about it. And I didn't do it. It's not that you didn't want to know. It's just . . . I don't know how to explain it. It was like another part of your life that's over. It's like it wasn't really you there. Think back and remember but it is like you think it was somebody else.

Like other survivors, Matthew is struggling with the meaning of survival. Of the children in the area who acquired acute lymphoblastic leukemia, only Matthew survived.

Why would God save me and not save somebody else in the same situation? Does that mean I have something to do in this world or does that mean I'm just lucky? That's the part I always still think about today. I still question that today.

Matthew has "never talked about this before except to myself. It seems like there is something I'm supposed to be doing in this world, but I don't know what it is. There is this deep big feeling inside of me." Recently, he has wondered whether the answer might lie in his new relationship.

Every time I have gotten into a relationship or whatever, I have never necessarily wanted to get married. I've come close but it just wasn't right. It didn't feel right. Because it feels like I'm supposed to be doing something else. But, I look at the situation where I'm with my girlfriend now. We've spent a year and a half, almost 2 years, [together] and she has two kids. And I love them. Maybe that's what I am supposed to be. I mean, because their dad isn't their dad and maybe I am supposed to be their dad. You know what I mean? You have to think, "Why did I live? Was it luck? Was it the lottery?" Maybe it was just me.

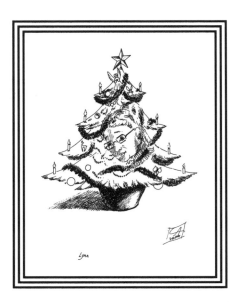

Lynn's Remembrance of Her Grandmother

7

A Family Affair

Lynn's Story

> While we try to teach our children all about life,
> our children teach us what life is all about.
>
> —Angela Schwindt

Lynn is 18 years old, Caucasian, and lives with her family in a small town north of Pittsburgh. She has one brother, 4 years younger. Lynn is petite, only 4'11" in height, and has the solid, stocky build of a cheerleader. She has long, dark black, curly hair that falls below her shoulders; dark, deep brown eyes; and a smooth, clear, milky complexion.

Lynn graduated from high school and now attends a small college in northwestern Pennsylvania. She is an elementary education major because "I always liked kids and I am good around them." Lynn devotes all of her energies to college; the courses that involve reading are very difficult for her and she spends all of her free time getting tutored.

Lynn was very quiet during the interview. She seemed reticent, almost uncomfortable, about talking of her experiences and would provide few details about her illness, her hospitalization, or her return to school. To make her more comfortable, Lynn's mother, who was waiting outside, was invited to join the discussion, "She understands what I've been through and I don't have to talk about it . . . she just knows." The strong relationship between mother and daughter was clearly apparent in the glances, smiles, clenching hands, and even tears that the two of them shared during the interview. As Lynn's mother put it,

The whole experience deeply created a strong bond between Lynn and myself. I can look at her eyes and just know what she is thinking or feeling . . . like if she's not feeling well . . . or if something is bothering her. We are part of each other [in the physical sense], of course, but we are also part of each other's souls. This experience made us part of each other emotionally and spiritually. We don't discuss it. It just exists.

ONSET OF THE DISEASE AND TREATMENT

It was in November 1981 when Lynn started to have flulike symptoms. She was 6 years old. "I remember [lying] on the couch and I was feeling really bad and [my parents] didn't know what was wrong." Her mother recalls,

It was right around Thanksgiving when we first started to notice that she must have the flu. She was achy, and tired, and she had a fever. I hadn't taken her to the doctor; I was just treating her with Tylenol. We just thought it was the flu and that was all.

Then, Lynn started complaining that her legs were hurting. "[They] hurt so bad, she couldn't walk. She started crawling around." That prompted her parents to take Lynn to the family doctor.

This was about a week and a half after she started getting sick. He [the family doctor] did a little bit of testing. I think he suspected it was [leukemia] right away, [but] we still really didn't have any idea. He wanted us to go to an oncologist in town and have some further testing done. So we went . . . right the next day. He did the testing and he said he wanted to put her in the hospital for more testing. I still was making no connection with leukemia.

Lynn was taken to the closest hospital, where a tentative diagnosis was made.

After all the testing was done, the doctor came into the room. My husband and I were there, and my father. Here I was thinking the doctor would just come in and say Lynn needs an antibiotic or something. Instead, [he] blurted out that Lynn had leukemia. Well, they don't realize people are not prepared to hear something that. It was an incredible experience at the time. I was watching myself in slow motion thinking they were telling someone else this news and not me. All I remember thinking is, "This is fatal."

Lynn was transported by ambulance, immediately, to Children's Hospital and was admitted on December 20, 1981. Her left leg was tender, swollen, and warm. Her tonsils were enlarged. She was pale, anxious, and tearful. CBC (complete blood count) blood work and a bone marrow biopsy confirmed that Lynn had acute lymphoblastic leukemia. But they had caught it early; a spinal tap found no leukemic cells in the spinal fluid. Chemotherapy treatments began immediately. "They [the physicians at Children's Hospital] explained that their main goal was to get her right into remission . . . as soon as possible."

Induction therapy lasted from December 20, 1981, until February 10, 1982, although Lynn was discharged from the hospital on December 31, 1981, and continued the treatments at home or on an outpatient basis. Her chemotherapy regime consisted of vincristine, L-asparaginase, and methotrexate. From January 1, 1982, to February 10, 1982, CNS prophylaxis was added—1,800 CGY of radiation to the head area. In addition, Lynn took antibiotics. During the second phase of treatment, the intensified treatment phase, Lynn was introduced to the drug 6-MP, and she was invited to enter an experimental treatment protocol.

Some of the children would be on medication for 3 years and some for 5 years. The doctors wanted children off chemotherapy by 3 years and they were trying to see if they would get the same results [with the shorter treatment]. The longer you are on chemotherapy the more side effects you can have. So, we chose for Lynn to be part of the protocol. She would be one of the children who would be off chemotherapy in 3 years. Of course they said if Lynn started to regress, they would immediately put her back on chemotherapy. Then they started her on the medication and I thought, "Did we make the right decision?"

Maintenance therapy lasted until April 12, 1985. The entire treatment regime took a little more than 3 years.

LYNN'S REACTIONS TO THE DIAGNOSIS AND TREATMENT

Lynn wouldn't talk much about the early days in the hospital. "I was in the hospital a couple of weeks in the beginning. Then, [after I was discharged], I received chemotherapy and radiation together." But she did remember losing her hair. "I remember losing my hair at Christmas. I remember it was Christmas time . . . [because] they got me a tree. Santa Claus came while I was there and there were a lot of presents, but I was really too sick."

Lynn knew she was very sick, but she was not told at the time that that she had cancer. "I don't remember them [my parents or the doctors] telling me. No. They never told me. I always just thought I had a very bad cold or something that was making me very sick like a bad flu." But over the next several years, as her level of understanding increased, her parents informed her bit by bit. "They started telling me a little by the age of 10 or so." Lynn thinks this was a wise approach. "I think kids are too young to understand what's going on, and maybe they would become more frightened."

Lynn did not develop any really close relationships during her stay at the hospital. "I had a private room at the hospital, so I didn't make any friends. But what stands out in my memories is that the doctors were very gentle and always looking out for me." She passed the time by "coloring and stuff like that. Watched TV and read books." But there were "bad parts, too, like the spinal taps and the bone marrows. They were really a lot of pain. I was crying a lot. I always had a teddy bear to hold for comfort." She also had her mother to hold on to. "My mom stayed with me mostly during the treatments. . . . I remember somebody being there all the time."

IMPACT ON THE FAMILY

Lynn's illness had a profound impact on her family. On first hearing of the diagnosis, Lynn's mother was devastated. "I just ran out of the room. I had to think. Well, back then, cancer wasn't as far as it is now with treatment." But she had to adjust quickly, because the burden of dealing with Lynn's illness fell mostly on her shoulders.

I would stay the entire week with Lynn; I slept on a cot in her room. He [Lynn's father] stayed at home during the workweek. Then he'd come a lot on the weekends to relieve me for a few hours while I went home to collect my emotional self. Then I would return.

Lynn thought the arrangement was great. "I remember them both staying with me at different times. I remember somebody being there all the time. I was never alone." But it took its toll on Lynn's mother.

It was all on me during that time. I talked to the doctors and nurses. I handled seeing Lynn hurting every day and trying to comfort her. It was me that was trying to learn the medical stuff. Even when she came home and was getting treatment, it was me who was home all day handling everything. It was hard on me.

And it was hard on Lynn's parents' relationship, as well. "We had a problem because my husband thought I would handle everything. He thought he was doing his part just by going to work every day."

And to make matters even worse, the family had problems with the insurance company. Lynn's father was a buyer and had just changed jobs when Lynn was diagnosed with ALL.

There was a problem at the time with Lynn being covered by insurance because my husband had just switched jobs. He thought his insurance would cover things. We thought since he [had] started to work there, it would all be on his insurance. [But] they said that she wasn't under their policy at the time [of diagnosis]. You know, we had to go through this whole big process with the insurance company. After a battle, they accepted it. We were fortunate in the end: the company he was working for went to bat for him when they found out how sick Lynn was. It was just another problem to deal with among many that we really didn't need.

Lynn's illness was also hard on her little brother. In the early stage, with Lynn's mother at the hospital all the time, Lynn's brother was sent to stay with his grandparents.

My son was a toddler at the time. I think he was 2 or 3 years old. He went and stayed with my mom. I remember she had his Christmas and his birthday for him because I was involved with Lynn at the hospital.

As Lynn's recovery progressed, and the family was reunited at home, her brother was often confused by how their parents dealt with the two of them. "He'd get mad when he was punished for something he did, [and] Lynn didn't get punished for what she did. It's hard raising a healthy child and at the same time trying to raise a sick child."

But the impact on the family went deeper than these remembered incidents. Lynn's mother summarized it well.

No one fully understands . . . what something like this can do to a family. Everything just stops in its tracks. You don't go forward and you can't go backward either. You simply exist day to day on raw emotion. Everything that you knew your life to be . . . the familiarity and security . . . no longer exists. It's gone forever. . . . Things are never the same again.

You know what true fear is and you realize how really vulnerable you and your family are to things that are out of your control. You want to protect your child from bad things happening to them and getting cancer is almost a slap in your face, as if to say, "Who are you kidding?" And for the first time you recognize that you can't protect your child from everything that happens on this earth. Then you feel helpless and guilty for bringing them into such a world and exposing them to pain and suffering while knowing you can't protect them from all the harm that exists out there.

To make matters for the family even more complex, Lynn's maternal grandmother was diagnosed with lymphoma (a form of cancer) approximately a year after Lynn had been diagnosed. Lynn was still going through treatments at the time.

They [Lynn's parents] told me my grandmother got sick. It was my mother's mother. It was about a year after I became sick. She had the same thing that I had but it was a form of cancer that they couldn't help. Only a few months after being sick, she died.

Lynn's mother remembers the time, vividly.

My mother became ill almost at the end of the first year of Lynn's battle with cancer. It happened around May and June of 1981. Lynn had been sick in December of 1980 and began treatments at the end of December and the beginning of January of 1981. It was like Lynn started improving and my mother started getting sick. It was really sad and [a little] eerie, too. You see, my mother was a very religious woman and she used to pray every day for Lynn that it would be her *that would have the cancer and not Lynn . . . that God should take* her, *not Lynn. Do you think her prayers came true? God spared my daughter but took my mother.*

Lynn feels guilty about surviving an illness that her grandmother did not survive. She was very close to her grandmother and "never quite got over everything that happened. It was really too much." And Lynn maintains a strong connection to her grandmother to this day. "She had given me a little Christmas tree for my hospital room. I had just been diagnosed and was starting the treatments. I still put that Christmas tree up in my bedroom today . . . 12 years later."

Lynn's mother has always been very protective of her. "She [Lynn's mother] would watch a [TV] program about cancer or something, and she wouldn't let me watch it. She would see people dying, and she wouldn't let me see that." Lynn's mother "didn't want her to think she had even a chance of dying." Lynn's mother had understood from conversations with the doctors and nurses that she was not to let Lynn

see you get emotional. [They were told that] if we walked into the room upset, she'd see it in our eyes. They said it would have a big effect on her if she saw signs in us of being upset. It would affect how she would react to the medicine. So we'd pull ourselves together, as we would go into her room. It was really hard to do that.

Two things helped Lynn's mother get through this time. First, being included in discussions with the doctors, and being allowed to stay with Lynn during her treatments and overnight in the hospital, were a great comfort. "Children's Hospital always let the parents be a part of everything. I was able to stay right in her room with her. I had a cot right there." Second, she found a friend.

We met due to circumstances, and yet it was like I knew her for a long time. Her daughter had been diagnosed with leukemia, maybe 4 or 5 years before Lynn was diagnosed. Our daughters had gone to the same school and, do you believe, both had been diagnosed with leukemia. Her daughter was 4 or 5 years older than Lynn was. She [the other child's mother] had found out about Lynn from one of her friends. She told this other person that if I ever needed anybody to talk to, to call her. Well, I did call her, which shows my own desperation at the time. She helped me tremendously. It's just you have somebody to talk to that is outside all of this but still has understanding of you and the whole situation. Instead of simply listening to doctors [and being told] this is how it's going to be . . . you actually have someone to talk to . . . a person who has gone through this and made it. So, I would call her all the time . . . just to compare what Lynn would be going through at that time. She supported me. She'd say, "She's going to get through this right now. It's going to get better. This is normal what she is experiencing."

Then, a few years later, Lynn's mother had the opportunity to reciprocate.

A neighbor who lives next door to my father has a grandson who was diagnosed with leukemia. I found out about it and called her. I told her if she ever wanted to talk to me just call me. She did and we've talked a lot. It really does help. It's sort of a rippling thing: one person helps another person and then they help someone else. The circle goes on.

TREATMENT SIDE EFFECTS

Lynn had many of the usual side effects of chemotherapy: bloating, hair loss, headaches or nausea following treatments, and stunted growth. For example, from early on in the treatment regime, Lynn developed "a really round face and big stomach." Lynn's mother added,

Her personal features became distorted to us. As a mother, to see your child like that, with no hair, a pudgy, round face, and a fat protruding stomach, you have to remind yourself it is only temporary while the doctors use the drugs to help her get better. Still, it pulls at your emotions at the time. It is a constant reminder that everything is not all right. You ask yourself, "Where is my beautiful healthy baby girl?"

Lynn also lost her hair.

I decided not to get one [a wig]. I thought they were for older people. So, I just wore a scarf, sometimes. My mom says that I never wore it around her. But around my grandparents, I would wear the scarf and then take it off when I felt comfortable.

When her hair grew back, the color and texture were different. "It was darker and curly. They said something at the time that maybe the chemotherapy affects the hair pores. The doctors used to call it 'the new and revised chemo hair treatment.'"

Headaches were a routine aftereffect of the spinal taps. "They were really bad headaches where she would actually throw up."

Finally, Lynn did not grow very tall. Lynn's doctors estimated that, in the absence of medication, she might have grown 3 to 4 inches taller than her current 4'11". But to Lynn, being short is "no big deal. It's not something I dwell on much. It doesn't take any enjoyment out of living for me." And her mother adds,

We didn't lose her, so what's the big deal as to whether or not she could have been taller? That person is important, not their hair or height. . . . You have to keep your priorities in perspective after you've made it through this ordeal. You don't think, well, her hair could have been different, or she could've been taller. It just isn't important. Life is important.

In addition to the standard side effects, an unexpected additional side effect was the appearance of temper tantrums. The doctors had mentioned that the medications might lead to temper tantrums, but Lynn and her family were unprepared for the sudden and unpredictable outbursts.

You couldn't prepare for one because you didn't know when one was going to happen. It was living on the edge. She would get so . . . frustrated. One day, she ripped curtains off the rod on the wall. Another [time] she was just sitting there with her brother, and she got mad, and she just slapped him. And, of course, he didn't know what was going on and he would get upset. Then I'd have two children upset, frustrated, and crying. And I'd get frustrated, too. It was so upsetting at the time. It put a strain on our family.

Lynn, herself, did not remember much of her behavior at that time.

It's very vague in my memory. I can't really say what I was feeling or what I did when I had a tantrum. I know I had them, but I can't give any details about it. Maybe that's a good thing. I'd probably feel bad about . . . giving my mother such a hard time.

THE SCHOOL EXPERIENCE

Lynn was diagnosed in December 1980 while she was in kindergarten in a Catholic elementary school. She was tutored at home by her mother

when she was too sick to attend school; the school did not offer homebound instruction.

The teachers just gave the papers to me and then I had to decipher what to do. I was not a
teacher so it was sometimes hard knowing what to do, how to do it, or what to expect from
Lynn academically especially while she was going through all this painful stuff.

When it was time to return to school, Lynn's mother made sure that the
school was aware of Lynn's medical condition.

I think they [teachers] really need to know things, so I was the one that let the teachers
know about Lynn's condition. We talked about what to do if there was like an outbreak of
chicken pox . . . or something. I do feel I educated the teachers. I don't think they knew much
about leukemia.

At first, her advice wasn't taken seriously, and Lynn's second-grade teacher
started out by treating Lynn as she would everyone else. "I remember telling
the teacher I had a headache and she said to me, 'Okay. You'll be fine.'" The
teacher was supposed to call Lynn's mother and alert the school nurse. She
did neither. "Then I got real sick. I threw up and everything." Lynn's mother
was very angry.

Sometimes you lose your patience with people who seem like they are not listening to what
you are trying to tell them. . . . I don't know . . . maybe she thought Lynn was faking it.

After that first incident, the school "would call me about every little
thing, even if she fell and scratched her knee or something." But Lynn
never took advantage of her condition. "After that day, the school nurse
would always ask me if I had a headache. I never faked it. I was pretty honest about those things. I don't feel I ever used my illness to get out of school
and to be home."

When the dreaded chicken pox outbreaks occurred "the school would
always let me know and I would keep her at home." But even these precau-
tions were not enough to keep her from eventually succumbing to the virus.

I called the doctor about the outbreak at school. I took her into the office and he gave her a
shot. But she got really sick with the chicken pox. They looked really bad on her body. We
had to watch her all the time. Lynn got them worse than a healthy child. Also, she got a high
fever. It was really scary at the time. If I remember correctly, chicken pox is a virus and with
her immunity system so low while having chemotherapy, it just made it worse for her. I'd

heard it can even be life threatening for a child who has cancer. But the doctors seem to know exactly what to do.

Lynn's classmates at school knew she was sick but since Lynn was in kindergarten, they certainly did not understand the seriousness of her illness. The kindergartners sent her pictures or cards, and they said a prayer for her every morning in school.

I would say that her friends at school really didn't know that much. They never knew how ill she really was at the time. They were too young to truly understand. I think the parents knew about it . . . but the kids themselves, I don't think they really did.

Lynn never tried to hide her condition.

When she did go back to school, she had a butch haircut . . . because she lost all her hair. Lynn did wear a scarf one day . . . when she was being tested as to whether she should go on to first grade. Then when it came September, she just went without the scarf. She never said anything and I didn't bring it up. Lynn was at a point by that time where no hair was acceptable to her. She didn't think anything about it.

And Lynn's mother and father never talked to her about her illness, the side effects, or the problems they might be causing her in school

. . . because [we] never wanted her to think she was any different. I didn't want her to have something else to worry about. I didn't want to say to her, "Well, are any of the kids making fun of you?" Because I didn't want her to think they were supposed to be making fun of her.

Lynn never really wanted people to know about her illness. She was afraid that they would treat her differently if they knew she was ill or had cancer. So, on advice from her mother, she did not tell her friends until long after the treatments had been completed. Her mother pointed out that

they didn't treat her differently because she told them [about her illness] when she was already okay. But I feel that if she had told them she was actually sick, and they would have seen how sick she really was, they would have treated her differently.

Of course, there were exceptions. "My best friend knew about the leukemia and she didn't treat me any differently." And the secrecy caused problems for her.

I remember when she was in sixth grade when she got her wish from Make-A-Wish. She could have some guests or friends participate in her wish fulfillment. Her friends didn't

know about [what this was all about] and she kind of wanted to keep it that way. But yet,
she wanted them to be there for her. She didn't know quite what to do.

When she started to tell others about her illness, it was very difficult. "I had a boyfriend at the time. . . . It was hard telling him. I cried, and he just held me. I was uncomfortable about the subject. But [my friends] were very comforting."

AREAS OF SCHOOL DIFFICULTY

Lynn's mother did not want her daughter to repeat kindergarten or any subsequent grade; she wanted Lynn to stay with the classmates she knew before she became sick. And the school seemed satisfied enough with her progress. "They never said to hold her back in any year in elementary school. She always got As, Bs, and Cs. She never did get really bad grades." But, beginning in second grade, the school did schedule Lynn for remedial services because they recognized some learning difficulties.

Lynn did have difficulty in reading and math after treatments. She was always in remedial groups for math and reading. Since she attended a Catholic elementary school, Lynn was separated from her class and had to go to a van outside school to get remedial help.

And these remedial services have certainly colored her memories of school.

I feel they sort of isolated me. I remember feeling left out. I'd come back to the classroom after being tutored and the kids would be doing something I missed out on. So, either I missed the activity entirely or I was always playing catch up.

And, as a result, Lynn's mother now has second thoughts. "Maybe she would have done better had she gone through kindergarten again . . . just to, you know, make her a bit further ahead. I don't know . . .

Throughout school, in her Catholic elementary school and her public high school, Lynn experienced problems in reading comprehension, sequencing her thoughts correctly in written expression, and concentration or attention. "There is a definite learning problem with comprehension. I know this because of all the tests she took to get in [remedial classes]. You could see comprehension was always low." Her spelling and math were considered average.

Lynn could work with numbers okay, but when it was a story problem and required read-ing and comprehending, she had problems. If a problem was written out [in math symbols], she could do it. But when it was in the form of a reading problem, she had a hard time fig-uring it out. She [also] had trouble with real-life math problems like dealing with the store.

And handwriting was a problem. Lynn uses "a different finger, my ring finger, in controlling the pencil in handwriting. That's why I have a bump on it right here."

The seriousness of these problems was not really reflected in her grades. "In elementary school I had Bs and in high school I had like a C av-erage. But my reading was always low." To accomplish these grades, Lynn and her mother had to work very hard. "My mom would always go over it [the schoolwork] with me whenever I needed help in a subject." And what surprised them both was that no one had prepared them for the school problems.

The doctors never discussed that there might be some kind of problems in learning after the treatments. They just talked about the sickness . . . throwing up . . . and the headaches. I feel they should tell the parents of at least the possibility. It would relieve some of the parents' burden. Then if the parents know of something, they could get help right off the bat for their child. They could've done something about it . . . right then and there.

Lynn's learning difficulties persist as she struggles through college.

It is very hard to get my thoughts in order. I have trouble getting my thoughts in sequen-tial order when I go to write something on paper like an answer to something in a para-graph, or writing a report. My reading is really low, [especially] in comprehension. I find college really difficult.

But Lynn is not shy about asking for help. "There are special services at college, like the Comprehension Workshop that I go to. [The teacher] gave me books to read and exercises to do. I have a tutor at college, too."

Lynn never had anyone in school to talk to about the emotional overlay of her illness, and, in retrospect, she missed that. "You need somebody that is there if you need to talk. I never shared my emotions with my teachers. I only would ask the teacher what the class knew; that was my coping strategy."

Lynn's mother also found Lynn's school years very difficult.

I talked to the teachers, principal, and the school nurse. It was left up to me. I am no teacher and I am no doctor. It would have been better if the teachers and school nurse could have heard things from a doctor. I think the school should have a connection with the doctor or someone from the hospital to prepare them a little bit for what might happen or what to expect.

I found myself assuming roles that I had no preparation for. It was difficult. I was Lynn's tutor at home and yet I was not a teacher. I was Lynn's doctor administering medication at home and learning medical terms as well as communicating with the school about Lynn's medical condition. It would have been a lot less stressful and demanding if I could have simply been Lynn's mother.

SURVIVING

Lynn has a quiet approach to life. She is not eager for excitement; she doesn't like to try new things. She is conscientious about her health. "Once a year I ago for a checkup and I get very nervous." And, she just wants to accomplish what she has set out to accomplish: finishing college and becoming a teacher. She thinks of herself as "conservative, reserved, and serious," and "looking at her today, you would never know what she went through at that time. We call her our miracle child."

Lynn would like to put the cancer experience behind her, but it is always with her.

Whenever I am not feeling myself, or get the flu, or something, there is a part of me that starts to wonder, "Am I sick again?" It's something you can't help. It is part your thinking and feeling. . . . It was a part of you . . . or rather it is a part of you . . . maybe one never really gets over it.

Lynn's mother has the same feelings of cancer paranoia.

Even today, when she says, "My leg hurts," I will get a panic attack. I guess it should be the person who had cancer who should get the attacks, but I am proof that the parents can have cancer paranoia, too. Any little ache, cold, flu, fever, scratch, anything, my mind mentally jumps and my heart speeds up with the thought, "Is it back?" I suppose we have a legitimate reason to feel that way. Cancer is sneaky, you know.

Lynn is not a deeply religious person, and she is "introverted, quiet; I don't talk much about my feelings." But the death of her grandmother to cancer while she, herself, was fighting the disease and surviving, has deeply affected her.

I get upset about my grandmother. I heard she had prayed to God every day when I had gotten sick. She prayed that God would take her instead of me . . . and He did. I wish both of us could have survived. I get real sad when I think about her. It stays inside me and follows me everywhere.

Lynn believes that there was a trade-off with God. God took her grandmother in her place. "Now, I have to handle what is the reason I was left here? What is my purpose here?" It is a question that haunts her. Her answer, at least for now, is

I believe that I have survived a tragedy . . . with my grandmother, my family, and myself. I believe life is just "simple" after that. I have a quiet and peaceful approach to life. When you go through something so big, it makes everything else so small and not worth getting so upset over. My goal with my life is to help children because . . . I enjoy them . . . I like working with them. Maybe that is why I am here. Maybe I'll be able to give something to a child because of who I am . . . and God knew that then, and now.

8

Keep Your Head
Up and Smile!

Ruth's Story

An optimist has a reason to smile, and
his smile reveals his faith in life.

—Unknown

Ruth is 25 years old and Caucasian. She is the youngest of four children—
one brother and two sisters. Her blond hair is styled in a pixie cut, and she
is only 5 feet tall. Ruth currently works in retail at a local chain store. She
was cheerful, outgoing, and open during the interview as she told her extraordinary story.

Ruth was diagnosed with ALL at the age of 7, at the end of the first grade
in May 1978, and her treatments lasted just over 2 years. Maintenance therapy ended in September 1980 when she was considered in remission. Then,
7 years later, at age 14, the cancer returned. This time the doctors decided
that she needed a bone marrow transplant. Each of her siblings was tested
for bone marrow compatibility but, unfortunately, none matched. In the fall
of 1986, she pulled through an autologous bone marrow transplant, then returned to and completed high school, and then attended Clarion College. It
was at college that she was diagnosed with a learning disability. Ruth graduated with a BA in History and Political Science. She reports that to this day
she has learning difficulties in mathematics, concentration, and reading
comprehension. Other residual problems include scarring of her scalp and
forehead, poor resistance to infection, endocrine problems, and infertitity.

Ruth's parents came with her to the interview. At the conclusion of the interview, they came into the room. They appeared grateful for an opportunity to share their memories, thoughts, and feelings concerning Ruth's illness because it had affected the entire family. Their comments are interwoven within Ruth's story.

ONSET OF THE DISEASE AND TREATMENT

Ruth's life trauma began at the age of 7 when she couldn't shake a head cold. She was at the end of her first-grade year in school. She had two admissions to the hospital for fever and night sweats but each time she was given antibiotics and sent home. She recalled her physical symptoms at that time.

I was having night sweats. I would wake up and be just soaked. I would have a low-grade temperature during the day, like between 98 and 100 degrees. And then at night it must have gone up at some time and then it would just break and I would be soaked. I literally would have to have my sheets changed. It started out of the blue. But I had this cold too that just wouldn't go away. It was constant. And eventually they found a virus. My gums would ache. I had a sore on my head that would drain, which they considered this virus thing. It just wouldn't heal. I had a blood test at our local hospital in Butler. Then I was sent to Children's Hospital in Pittsburgh where [they said] I had anemia. [The doctor] did blood tests and within 2 weeks he knew what it was. I would say the problems started at the end of February 1978 through the spring. I was finally diagnosed in May 1978 with acute lymphocyctic leukemia.

Ruth's parents interjected their memories of this time. They highly complimented Children's Hospital and the doctors. They also expressed believed sincerely that God had a hand in getting them to the right hospital and the right doctors.

When we took her to the family doctor, that is when they said she was anemic. And then at Butler Hospital, the doctor there said there is a virus in her blood. We thought well this doesn't make sense. It just wasn't registering. And again, here we are thinking we have to find somebody who knows what they are doing.

So the parents, themselves, called Children's Hospital and were seen within 2 weeks.

We said, "Doctor, what do you think here?" He said, "Well I'm 99% sure she has leukemia." He said we'll put her in Children's Hospital and the next day do a bone mar-

*row. He said we'll find out for sure. We had the best in Pittsburgh. We had no idea at
the time. It was like God said, "Hey, call this guy." We just felt God directed us all the
way through.*

Children's Hospital admitted Ruth and began the lengthy treatment
process. The induction phase began on May 5, 1978, and consisted of al-
lopurinaol and intrathecal methotrexate. A new ALL protocol was
started and Ruth received one dose of vincrinstine weekly, prednisone
daily, and L-asparginase every other day starting on the third day. She
was also administered the chemotherapy agents adriamycin and cytoxan. Ruth's cranial irradiation treatments were from June 12 through
June 27, 1978. She received 12 treatments to the head area with each dose
of radiation consisting of 2,400 cGy.

Maintenance therapy began on July 7, 1978, and continued through
September 15, 1980. The chemotherapy medications given during this
period at various intervals were vincristine, prednisone, adriamycin,
6-MP, cyclophosphamide, intrathecal methotrexate (given at the beginning of every cycle—every 84 days), and oral methotrexate. Ruth was
subjected to numerous bone marrows and spinal taps during the induction and maintenance stages of her therapy. Her entire treatment protocol lasted just over 2 years.

RUTH'S REACTIONS TO DIAGNOSIS AND TREATMENT

Ruth's memories of her treatment process appear not to have faded
with time.

*I remember I went into the hospital on my sister's 16th birthday. When I first started, I had
12 radiation treatments to my head. After that it was basic chemotherapy treatments,
spinal taps, bone marrows, all of those, which of course caused a lot of sickness, illness, and
irritability . . . and those lovely things that go along with it.*

Ruth also remembers how the doctors slowly weaned her off of the
chemotherapy over a 2-year period.

*When I first got sick I was down there [at the hospital] once a week for like so many months.
And then they got me into remission, and then it got to the point where I was going down
[to children's] to get treatment like once a month. Then slowly everything just kinda leveled
off and they eventually just took me off after 26 months of treatment, which was like 2
years. They then considered me cured.*

Now Ruth's parents had a decision to make.

She was on a 3-year program. And one day they [the doctors] confronted us with a study out of England that children did not do any better if they were on a 3-year program or a 26-month program. They said it was up to us [whether she continued on chemotherapy or stopped it then and there]. We said, "Hey take her off. Why put her through all that hell and everything?" So we thought why should she go any longer because that stuff is bad on the body. So we just took her off.

Unfortunately, after 5 years almost to the month of Ruth's last treatment for leukemia, she relapsed with the same form of leukemia—acute lymphocytic leukemia. Ruth was 14 years old and about to go into the ninth grade in school. It was the summer of 1985.

They brought me in with mononucleosis. Mono and leukemia are very close [to each other] in cells. They thought I had mono. Well, in fact I did have mono. My immune system was down and I caught mono. I had all the same symptoms again, the night sweats, the swollen glands, but they thought that it might be from the mono. I also had a plantar wart which [was similar] to when I had a sore on my head that wouldn't heal the first time. With my wart, it was like a sign . . . I had gotten a plantar wart and eventually mono and then they put me in and the cells just didn't look right. And that is when they realized that I had relapsed. It was hard to tell being that they were dealing with the mono also. It turned out to be ALL.

Ruth's mother took the relapse badly.

When my daughter suffered the relapse, I suffered an emotional relapse. The six of us [Ruth, her siblings, and her parents] came through this once before. This time it was a lot harder. I just didn't adjust to it well the [second] time and I am not proud of it.

Ruth went into treatment immediately.

Actually everything went well as far as I remember after the second diagnosis. They got me back in remission again very quickly, treated me for a year with chemotherapy and no radiation this time. I think I had a spinal tap every 3 months. They cut out the bone marrow tests . . . I didn't have to have the bone marrows every two months. I did have the methotrexate and vincristine, which is what I had before but I didn't have the real powerful sickening drugs. . . . I had to stay out of the sun with the methotrexate. There were just little side effects. Actually, of course, you lose your hair, which is normal.

Preparation for the bone marrow transplant was grueling. First, the physicians harvested Ruth's bone marrow by withdrawing a portion of it from her hipbones and purging it of any residual leukemic cells. Then came "8 days of hell," 4 days each of chemotherapy and total body radiation to destroy her remaining bone marrow before the cleaned marrow was reinfused a week later.

I went through a period where it was 4 straight days of total body irradiation and 4 days of chemotherapy. The drug they gave me was wicked. I got that the first 4 days and I got the radiation for the next 4 days. It was the total body irradiation. You were to stand for 30 minutes in this "play" glass box and you got zapped from head to toe, front to back. I was so sick. I was throwing up everywhere and I was so tired. And the last day for some reason, I got this burst of energy and I stood the whole 30 minutes. I didn't take any breaks. They [the technicians] were laughing because they were saying that I was the first patient in history that had ever done that. I said, "Yeah, I know. I have to set records everywhere I go."

Then what followed was an 8 week hospital stay. Ruth was kept in isolation while the new marrow took hold and blood cell reproduction took place. Because Ruth's own marrow was used, rejection was not a problem, but infections could be. So Ruth was given antibiotics and transfusions. She describes some of the dragons she had to slay during this battle for her life.

My counts had all dropped, my white count, my red count, everything, which is not good. I remember this; it was Halloween. The doctor came in to do something with the artery because my blood pressure was real low. And once again, to throw humor in it, my sister and her friends came down from college. I am really sick and she comes with a scary mask on. I am screaming because there is some kind of monster in my room. It was funny and weird. Then they did a bronchoscopy where they shove down the tubes through your nose and throat and that is how they found out I had Legionnaire disease (Legionnella) which is a kind of pneumonia. I think for 2 weeks I was like in intensive care. I don't remember any of this. I like lost 2 weeks of my life in there. Then they moved me back because I became stable. I remember the doctors coming and saying to me, "Rutty, just hang in there a couple more days. I know your counts are going to come up." And boom, didn't he know it! Like within a day or two I had 2 white cells.

But the roller-coaster ride wasn't over. And the peaks and valleys were often within a moment's breath of each other.

Everyone was thrilled [about my white blood cells coming up]. And of course the next day I lost them. Then they came back up. This is normal. One day you could have five and next day none. Then I had three, and then after that they just started coming up.

TREATMENT SIDE EFFECTS

Ruth experienced transient and long-term side effects first from the chemotherapy and radiation, then from the bone marrow transplant. When discussing the side effects, she maintained an optimistic and humorous attitude.

The first thing you feel is the hair loss. Maybe it's vain but like I am losing my hair! Who cares about my health . . . I am going to lose my hair! I got hit with it [the hair loss] when I was 7 and kids do make fun of you. Then, at 14, it happened again. When I left school, I had hair. Then when I came back, I had no hair. My classmates were startled. The kids were standoffish at first. When people don't know what's wrong, they tend to shy away from you . . . they are afraid they might turn out that way or they're afraid they might do or say something wrong. Then they began to understand I was the same as them. Actually I did have a boyfriend, who was very good about everything, a super guy. He was super through it all. I had gotten used to the stares when I would go shopping with my boyfriend and some idiot would poke fun and say, "You're bald." I didn't care. I didn't wear scarves or wigs because it just was not me. My girlfriends would understand and just take me for what I am. Back then . . . at that time . . . girls would say, "My God I have a pimple." I would say, "Well, look, I have no hair."

Ruth's hair grew back, but she was left with other, more permanent, side effects of her treatments: hearing loss, brittle bones, and sterility.

I am hard of hearing. My left ear is shot to pieces. When I got the mono and leukemia together . . . the mono got into my ear and damaged [it]. I have water back up and everything and it has just gotten worse. It is very distressful. I mean, I don't like people coming up behind me and I can't hear what they say. It even gets worse when I get sick like have a cold. My bones are just brittle. I remember I fell on my tailbone and sprained it. I couldn't take gym for 2 weeks.

I cannot have children; I'm infertile. My organs are still good . . . [but] I have been through menopause.

Finally, as she was recovering from the bone marrow transplant, Ruth developed facial shingles.

Facial shingles is an infection. I looked like a burn victim. It took out all this [pointing to her right eyebrow], got in my eye. Just kinda screwed up my whole forehead. And, of course, at the time it was really devastating. You are 16, and look at your forehead. People complain about pimples, Ruth has facial shingles. I'm like, "Hey I'll trade you, please. I don't mind a little bit of acne." I ended up losing my eyebrow and eyelashes over that.

And that devastation cannot be put entirely behind her. "Okay . . . every morning when I get up, I have to draw this eyebrow on my face. . . . I still get depressed occasionally when it [the eyebrow] won't go on right."

IMPACT ON THE FAMILY

Ruth's family was "solid and affectionate" throughout her illness. "My family was great; if it was not for my whole family crew, I would be going nutzo." She remembers her father as a "happy guy" and her mother as constantly reminding her to "keep your head up and smile!" Ruth's mother was the person she would go to, to talk about problems like being made fun of at school. She remembers staying with her mother in her parents' bedroom while going through the treatments. But though they were supportive, there were stresses and strains.

It is hard to explain . . . it is like you have a family, there is me then there is the rest of the family and we are all like in total opposite spectrums because they can kind of help you deal with what you are going through but they can't know what you are going through because they are not you. And the same with them. There were days when they just couldn't figure out why I was being such a pain. And there were days when I couldn't figure out why my parents or my family was so stressed out.

Perhaps the greatest stress was around money.

My parents are great. I don't know how they did it with the bill collectors calling. . . . We had one guy, just calling and calling; he was an insurance guy. My parents would just call him and tell him . . . I mean what do you say? "My daughter's got leukemia. We have medical bills up the butt." I mean they were giving a little bit of money monthly [toward the insurance bill]. Well, one day, this guy would not get off the phone. We told him my mom was out grocery shopping and he said, "I'll wait until she comes home." And he wouldn't get off the phone. Finally my mother had to go . . . she was friends with this guy who ran the insurance place. And the guy got fired.

Ironically, Ruth came out of remission only 3 weeks after her father paid off all the bills from their first round with leukemia. Ruth's father worked two jobs to try to defray the medical costs. When the second bout of leukemia was diagnosed, his coworkers, community residents, and students from Ruth's high school sponsored numerous fund-raising events. Her mother recalls, "I was never bitter. Why us? I mean, why not us? I just want a cure so that other parents don't have to go through what we have."

Ruth could not help but compare herself to her sisters in physical appearance and popularity. Her sisters had what Ruth referred to as "normal school years." Hers, by contrast, were "abnormal" and "different" and to cope, she developed an "I-don't-care attitude" to protect herself emotionally and psychologically.

My sisters are gorgeous. My brother is good-looking. They are a gorgeous family. I mean [my older sister] would be the one who had eight dates for the weekend. And Ruthy would be sitting at home. They couldn't figure out why I wasn't getting asked out. But they had a normal high school and grade school life. In high school, they were hip. They were cheerleaders and my brother played baseball. I do admit I was homecoming queen. But even after that, I sat at home on the weekends. And I think . . . I don't know . . . maybe I am being paranoid but no one wanted to kind of go out because they were uneasy going out with the girl who was sick. They wouldn't know how to handle it. You know what I mean, it wasn't normal. [Giggles] I was abnormal, I admit it, I was different . . . I don't care.

Ruth's mother shared her memories of Ruth's battles with cancer.

I look back on it now, and I think I don't know how she went through it, or how any of us did. When they took us in the room to tell us what she had, I remember hearing my husband ask, "How long?" From that day on, I learned to think in firsts—first cheerleader, first date, and first boyfriend. I learned to ask, "How many firsts can I get?" Illness can either bring you together or tear you apart, so we did try to laugh a lot to take the pressure off.

THE SCHOOL EXPERIENCE

Ruth was diagnosed during the spring of first grade and was tutored at home during the final months of school that year.

When I was in the first grade, the teacher that had my brother and [older] sister, her brother played baseball with my brother. I mean she was a younger teacher and she was very good friends of the family. And she came out to tutor. I was tutored after I was diagnosed. Last two months of school [first grade] I was tutored.

She did return for the last day of school "because it was a half day. The doctors were like, 'yeah, she has her energy back she can go and sit for a half day because they had a little party and everything.'" Ruth's mother informed the first-grade teacher about Ruth's illness, and Ruth presumes that the teachers informed her classmates. "Basically everyone kind of knew. You have to fill out little medical forms and my mom would usually call the teacher at home and say this basically is what she can do and what she can't do."

One of the most important people to smooth Ruth's return to school, however, was her first-grade best friend.

She sat right beside me the whole time and she went around and told everybody that "Ruthy has leukemia and that is why she doesn't have any hair, so don't make fun of her." And she did that also in my catechism class.

When Ruth returned to second grade after the summer break, life was difficult.

A good example of this was a girl had a birthday party, I wasn't invited because her mother thought I was contagious. I remember this girl coming to me and saying "It's not that I didn't want to invite you, but I already had too many people that I had to invite." I was the only girl that wasn't invited. Well, I'm not bitter. I had a party and I invited her, so her mother probably felt this big [holding her thumb and forefinger close together].

Ruth also vividly remembers being teased at school.

Second grade through fourth grade [were bad] because those few years I was getting chemo and all that. Like I said it [being teased] wasn't so bad. I don't know I guess I kind of got used to it, you know. I mean there are bad days and you laugh it off or you go home and cry it off you know. My mother . . . Oh . . . I remember this one time this one boy would not stop teasing me. Once she (mother) was picking me up to take me to a doctor's appointment. And he started making fun of me in the lunch line. We were walking me down and getting me ready to go to lunch and this kid made some comment and I don't think he realized my mom was behind me. Oh boy, she turned around; she laid into him, and then the teacher laid into him. But you know what . . . you can't do anything about it because the parents are going to let their kids get away with that. You know what I mean, it all stems from the home. So, what are you going to do?

Ruth also remembers that her mother taught her to handle these annoyances with courage and spunk.

You had little twits that made fun of you and made fun of you on the bus and I would go home and cry. There were days I did not want to go to school. I just didn't want go. She [my mother] would literally drag me out of bed and get me dressed and say, "Go!" My mother, God bless her, always taught all of us to keep our heads up and smile. And that is something that I always . . . even in my devastation of having facial shingles and looking like Yoda, the guy from Star Wars, *I still kept my head up and smiled no matter what people said or what people did.*

Of course there were some high points in school.

I remember my second-grade teacher, it was really hot one day and I had my scarf on and I went up and asked her do you mind if I take my scarf off because I didn't want to offend anyone else. She looked at me, she like got tears in her eyes and she's like "No, you go and you do it." And I took off my scarf and it got to the point from then on no matter if I had hair or not or if it was just coming in, I never wore a scarf. I just got really brave and felt this is me.

Third grade went well. "My third-grade teacher was great, and she knew if I was having a problem understanding something. I liked school then." And fifth grade went well, too, but that was because "the fifth-grade teacher was real cool about things, if I was having problems. She was good friends with my mom, too."
Fourth grade was a different story, though.

Fourth grade got kind of tough because we started learning sciences and stuff like that. I started having difficulty with school . . . understanding. I remember I was shunned more. The teacher just wouldn't call on me and went all around the room even though I was waving my hand; I had to stand up. I also went through a bad time when I lost my hair. My teacher would literally make a spectacle of it like in front of the class and say, "Your hair looks real good, it seems like it is coming in." I think she was trying to be nice. There were days when I wasn't feeling well, and it intimidated me more when the teacher would bring it up in front of the [class].

She was uneasy with it, is what I am thinking. I just don't think she knew how to deal with it. She didn't understand; she thought I was trying to cop out. And she would always bring attention to anything that you don't have to bring attention to because it is no big deal.

Sixth grade was a particularly bad year.

My sixth-grade teacher told me [things only] once. [Often], I didn't understand an assignment and I did it wrong and she chewed me out in front of the class and then chewed me outside the class and told me just because I was sick doesn't mean that she had any sympathy for me. She used to harass me constantly because I couldn't do certain things and I never told my mom or my dad. And one of my friends that was in my class, she went home and told her mother. My mom wouldn't have known any of this. And her mother told my mom at this sixth-grade banquet. And my mom confronted me and said, "Why didn't you ever tell me this? Why didn't you tell me you were having problems?" And I said I was afraid to.

There was no help available for students like Ruth. There were no guidance counselors in the school.

It was hard because it is not like now you have these special schools, not that I am retarded or anything like that, but special help [is available] now where they are discovering this. Back then, they didn't care; they just kind of passed you on.

By the time Ruth got to high school and through the bone marrow transplant, she had come to hate school. "Those [high school years] were the bad years. I missed a lot of school from being sick and I always felt like I was trying to catch up. Talk about stress!"

Several incidents contributed to Ruth's distaste for school. Her teachers were not very sympathetic.

I remember right after my transplant [but before she was back at school full time], I went up to talk to somebody up at the high school. A teacher said, "Well, when are you coming back to school? You gotta come back sometime." And I'm thinking, WAIT A MINUTE, the more I thought about it I was thinking you didn't go through what I went through. You try going through what I went through. I almost died in there. I deserve a little time off. And anyway, I was being tutored. So, it wasn't like I was getting "free out-of-school." You know, like where do you get off? I am coming back for my junior year. I'll be back in high school.

And many teachers really didn't appreciate what she was going through.

To make a long story short and sum it all up in a sense, it doesn't help when you go to school and you've [got] somebody like on my case who you either get made fun of [by] or you are having problems understanding and the teacher can't understand why you can't understand. And that right there, just kind of turned me off toward going to school.

There is a lot of stress. And it sounds funny for a little 7- or 8-year-old to have stress, but it happens. As it is, you have enough things to worry about, but they [teachers] like to add pressures to the pressures. They didn't want to go through my parents and add pressure to them. They would [just] go through me.

Her teachers not only didn't understand her learning problems; they also didn't understand how surviving cancer changes you.

I had a friend who wanted me to come to speak to his biology class. The teacher was like, bring her in. Then, she found out my age and didn't want me to speak because she didn't think that 16-year-old cancer patients knew what they were talking about. She wanted an adult. This is what I'm talking about. That woman who didn't want me to speak looked at me like I was a little kid. But when you are a little kid going through cancer they expect you to just handle everything. [And then] teachers expect you to be just right back in there [she snaps her fingers] you know like everybody else.

Nor did they or her family really appreciate how difficult it was for her to return to school after her second bout with cancer.

I think it was harder, I mean I got hit the second time a lot worse. I mean you are at that point where you are trying to make that physical image. You are going into junior high; you've got these good-looking girls and guys. And the scariest thing was going back to the ninth grade, not having any hair, and not having any friends, and all I had was Jim [her boyfriend], waiting there for me. People didn't know what happened to me, people thought I moved because I sat out my fall semester of my ninth-grade year. Then I came back. But until kids started to find out what was wrong with me, they . . . were just as cruel as teenagers as they were [in grade school]. . . . 'Cause like I said, when you don't fit in. And like I said, the more people found out, it wasn't as bad . . . but . . . all those insecurities always stay with you. I'm still very insecure about my forehead (scars from facial shingles). If I meet somebody new, a lot of times I don't like people getting real close to me because of my head.

And throughout all the difficulties, Ruth's mom was there for her.

[My mom] tried to help me out the best that she could. She was always like my tutor. I mean, she knew when I was having a bad day or I was just like "ahhh I don't feel like doing it."

Ruth's grades were not exceptional but she did get through school.

[My grades] were decent . . . average. I wasn't a straight A student . . . Bs and Cs. I'll admit it. I got a couple of Ds. It was usually in math (giggles). There are certain things like math I am horrible at. I can do a little algebra. I can add. I can subtract. I can multiply and divide. The computation wasn't difficult; it was like the geometry . . . forget it!

Her strongest area was writing and she kept a journal during her illness.

I used to write, actually I used to keep diaries. And I wrote songs, and . . . I will pat myself on the back and say I am an excellent writer—I am very good at writing. I love to write. I used to write poems, still do, I write stories, journals, and things like that. [I kept] up through college. I kept a journal when I got sick. And I kept one through college and then I kind of lost track of that.

Ruth's mother viewed Ruth's schoolwork differently than she did that of Ruth's siblings. "Let's face it, I didn't ground her when she got a C like

I did with her sisters and brother. How could I? I just didn't know whether she'd make it to the fourth grade."

AREAS OF SCHOOL DIFFICULTY

Although Ruth was not diagnosed with a learning disability until her entrance into college, she has been told that her school learning problems were "something like dyslexia." Ruth has a lot of problems with reading including a very pronounced difficulty in reading numbers. These problems certainly affect her retail job.

I notice it when I write numbers down at work (retail sales clothing) and I will read it back to the customer [and notice that I wrote it wrong]. Or like I noticed the other day, someone wanted to buy something, and what we do over the phone is we take down your credit card number. I wrote it down and I read it back wrong to her. I know I wrote it down right, but I wasn't reading it correctly. I catch myself, but it is scary. I don't like that feeling.

Another of Ruth's problems is in concentration.

When I had that OVR [Office of Vocational Rehabilitation] test, they would read a set of numbers to me. I would listen but I'd get lost. They would ask me to repeat it or repeat it backward. And I couldn't do that.

Ruth also believes that her reaction time is slow; it takes her a long time before something "sinks in" and she needs lots of repetition.

I am kind of slow in the sense that . . . not that I am stupid or anything like that . . . a good example was one morning I was making breakfast. And I pulled something out hot, out of the microwave. It sounds funny but it took like three minutes to set in . . . that I pulled something hot . . . and I was holding it. It was like "Oh!" I burned myself. Slow like that. I don't move quickly.

And Ruth reported other problems, as well.

I tend to stutter a bit. I talk very fast. And, I am hard of hearing. My left ear is shot to pieces. The mono got into my ear and damaged it. And because of it I'm loud. I'm like, I can't hear myself.

Despite these problems, Ruth not only completed college, she actually enjoyed it.

Things like history, English, and writing interest me. But it is the physics and the sciences I just can't comprehend. And I am not the smartest thing when it comes to math or things don't click. A lot of times people say, "What is 25 and 82?" You know I can't . . . give me a calculator or give me a pen and I'll do it. Of course, some numbers like 40 and 25 I can put together and say that is 65. Is that right (giggles)?

Accommodations were made for Ruth's learning difficulties so she could graduate from college.

What they did was they substituted, instead of me having to take a language because of my hearing and my learning disabilities, which they found out through the test [at OVR]. Instead I took an African history course, a multicultural course, which is right up my alley. It is something I can understand.

But her learning difficulties have held her back.

Let's put it this way, if I were smart, I am not saying I'm not smart, but if I were gifted, I would be a doctor right now. I would be going to med school. Like I said, a lot of times I get very devastated and frustrated because there so many things I'd love to do but I just know, not that I'm trying to sound negative, but I just know I can't do it. Like chemistry floored me. I just couldn't do the math work.

Yet despite these frustrations, Ruth can still laugh at herself and at her problems. "The big joke was when I first learned how to drive. They would say, 'Ruthy turn left,' and I would get nervous or frustrated and go the other way." And she has never let her illness, the treatments, or the residual effects keep her from setting high goals for herself. While in high school Ruth became a cheerleader, was crowned homecoming queen, then graduated from high school, attended college, and graduated from college. It is no wonder that she won the St. Francis Health Foundation's Courage to Come Back Award for her determination to beat the odds.

SURVIVING

Ruth believes that the illness and its treatment, and the resulting psychological stress have had a profound effect on her life. For one thing, she missed out on some normal developmental experiences.

I think I am backward when it comes to dating. I think like a 16-year-old sometimes. I admit it. Like I said, I had friends and people I talked to on the phone, but I was always kind of the one who sat home on the weekends and didn't have any dates. I'd go to football games but I'd go by myself. It is almost like I became a loner. I was friends with everybody; I did-n't really click on. I was like that in college too. I wasn't in a sorority or anything because I didn't believe in them.

When she did start dating, Ruth "didn't know how to just go out and have fun because I was always looking for a relationship or something like that. My personal life, it kind of goofed things up."

Ruth has spent the past 10 years since her second remission feeling as though the events of her early life caused her to "miss out on something. I was backward, and backward as far as schooling and everything. I don't know if I will ever get that back."

Ruth is also very uncomfortable about her height. "Even now I see these tall beautiful women working in the mall down there. And you know there's me Miss Five Foot. I'm five feet tall!" And she feels very insecure.

Let me give an example. When I met my boyfriend, he was an auto manager at Mont-gomery Ward. The lady I worked for, she is extremely attractive. She is 31, and 5'10", and has the longest legs you'd ever seen. She is beautiful. And I still ask Ed to this day, "What did you see in me?" because he is extremely attractive. And he said, "I just liked your com-pany more." And I'm like well I don't know [laughter], what are you doing with me? I don't know what it is. It is something that always sticks with you.

Ruth's experience with illness has made her want to do things for other people. She greatly admires a college friend of hers, Jay, who had stomach cancer.

He had a great personality. At the time, he was in remission; that was about 3 years ago. He had the most positive attitude. He would go around and talk to the schools and colleges. I think that is the greatest thing.

Ruth feels it's significant for children to see young people who have made it through, who have been there and made it.

I would love to do something like that. If I could find a full-time job going out and explain-ing to people—to kids . . . not so much the grown-ups, but most especially the kids. You know having a little group therapy that way. A lot of times [kids] don't feel like talking but, you know, someone like Jay saying, "Hey, I know where you have been. I know there are days you feel like crap or you [are made to] feel insecure by the boy or the girl who is Mr. or

Miss Attractive. Or . . . when you feel intimidated about other things." Like I said, kids that
are sick need understanding.

Ruth also acknowledges the significant impact that the Make-A-Wish
Foundation had on her at the time of her illness. "I was in the fifth grade
and got a free trip to Florida through the Sunshine Foundation which is
now the Make-A-Wish Foundation. This is a great organization." She also
recognizes that this foundation has influenced her outlook on life.

*Someday, when I am rich and famous, I would like to open up my own ranch. I love horses.
I don't know how to ride. That is another thing, I want learn how to ride horses. I'd like to
have a ranch and have a weekend thing for these kids who are sick because all they see are
hospitals. Get them out and take like five families and stay at the ranch and be able to ride
horses and just have one hell of a ball for a weekend and just forget about everything. It
would be free of charge. And if they wanted to pay anything, it would go toward [cancer]
research. You gotta have money. You gotta be like Marlo Thomas to do these things. But it
is a long-term dream that I would like to do someday. It is more important to give than to
get. Giving is what makes us truly happy.*

Ruth does not think of herself as a typical 25-year-old because of what
she lived through as a child. "I look back now and think, 'How did I deal
with it?' I think experience-wise it has made me look at life much differently
than average 25 year olds." She believes she has "been to hell and back" and
that some people may think she has "an attitude."

*I am one of these (people) who likes to live life for today . . . do what you can. I don't know
what tomorrow is going to bring to me. If you have a dream, DO IT! There shouldn't be
anything stopping you. Life is too short to worry about it. I can't let things get me down.*

Ruth has certainly internalized the lesson drilled into her by her family.
"I've always been told to just keep your head up and smile. Keep your
chin up, kid. Once you think you've hit rock bottom, there is only one way
out, and that is up."

9

One of Life's Lessons

Joseph's Story

My disease has been a demanding teacher that has guided
me—sometimes with a heavy hand—toward what I need to do.

—Tom O'Connor

Joseph is a handsome, African American man, 20 years of age. He is tall
(approximately 5'10"), with deep brown eyes and a friendly, warm smile.
Joseph was a little hesitant to talk about his cancer experience; he reported
that "I have never shared those experiences with anyone" before this interview. He spoke cautiously, weighing his words carefully. It was obvious
that some of the memories were very painful. Joseph reported having had
very few difficulties in school either during or after the cancer, and he was
looking forward to attending college where he planned to study physical
therapy. He had high expectations for a successful future and expressed a
strong desire to "give back." While waiting to begin college, Joseph was
working at a chain pizza restaurant.

ONSET OF THE DISEASE AND TREATMENT

The cancer ordeal began when Joseph was 7 years old, in the second
grade, living with his mother in McKeesport, Pennsylvania.

One night I was just having a really bad headache and I had a real high fever. My eyes were burning. I couldn't like open my eyes. So my mom called a cab and she took me to the hospital over there. From there, you know, they were like checking me over and I think I blacked out on the table. And I woke up the next day at Children's [Hospital].

Joseph was diagnosed with acute lymphoblastic leukemia in December 1983. The Induction phase of his treatment lasted from December 14, 1983, to January 1, 1984. He remained in the hospital during that 2-week period, and although his mother was with him at the beginning, it was soon evident that "she just didn't have the strength" to see Joseph through the illness. A foster parent was assigned to him while he was still in the hospital. He remained hospitalized for the better part of the next 3 months. His doctors were concerned that "sending him home to live with his mother might lead to problems with compliance."

Chemotherapy continued with doses of prednisone for 28 days, vincristine and daunonycin once a week for 4 weeks, intrathecal cytarabine and intrathecal methotrexate two doses each, and L-asparaginase. He had a very good response with resolution of adenopathy (swelling of the lymph glands) and swelling of the spleen and liver. Joseph was also treated with triple antibiotics; his white blood cell count improved and the fever was resolved. His CNS showed no malignant cells.

Joseph's consolidation phase lasted from January 23, 1984, to February 7, 1984. The plan was to taper his prednisone slowly, to begin 6-MP orally daily, to give cytarabine as called for by his protocol on days 1–4, 8–11, and again on day 14, and to begin cranial irradiations. Joseph received cytoxan on day 0 and day 14 of the consolidation phase. He received intrathecal methotrexate once a week on days 1 and 8. His cranial (brain) irradiation began on January 24, 1984, and ended on February 6, 1984. Joseph had 10 treatments at 1,800 rads. He tolerated this stage of treatment extremely well. He complained of chills, a sore throat, diarrhea, much nausea, and vomiting. His white blood cell count fell slowly but was still within the acceptable limits. He began to show hair loss.

Joseph's maintenance treatments lasted for 84 weeks. They began on July 7, 1984, and ended on April 15, 1987. During this phase his chemotherapy consisted of methotrexate (12 mg a day), vincristine (1.5 mg by IV monthly), prednisone (40 mg five times monthly), and mercaptopurine (75 mg weekly). Throughout this period, Joseph lived with a foster family.

At the end of the maintenance phase, Joseph was given a bone marrow aspiration and a bilateral testicular biopsy was performed; both showed no remaining signs of leukemic cells. His entire treatment protocol had lasted 4 years.

Joseph had a follow-up office visit on March 7, 1994. He showed no evidence of leukemic cells. There were no complaints. He appeared to be sleeping and eating well. His records were signed off with "ALL has been cured!"

At the time of the interview, it had been 8 years since Joseph's last treatments and there had been no signs of any secondary forms of cancer.

JOSEPH'S REACTIONS TO DIAGNOSIS AND TREATMENT

At the time of diagnosis, Joseph did not understand the nature of his illness or the reasons he needed to stay in the hospital. "I think I was too young to understand." His mother tried her best to explain.

I asked her, "What am I doing here? I want to go home." And she was telling me, "Honey, you can't, you can't go home." I just remember her crying and trying to tell me what was wrong with me but she couldn't do it. Every time she went to tell me, she started crying and turned around and walked out of the room.

Explanations fell instead to Joseph's pediatric oncologist. It was the doctor who told 7-year-old Joseph what his illness was, and about his treatments and the necessary procedures like spinal taps and bone marrow aspirations that would have to be done to him. It was his doctor who supported and comforted him during this traumatic time.

Mom really couldn't explain it . . . "cause you know she was crying and . . . but he [the doctor] informed me. He told me before anything happened to me. He would stand there and explain it to me, "We are going to do this and it is going to happen this way." When I got my bone marrow and spinal taps and everything, he would show me the needle and show me the syringe. He did everything right in front of me and explained it to me what it was and what it was he was going to do to me. And that helped it go a lot easier.

Joseph remembered vividly the extreme and piercing pain he experienced from the procedures such as the spinal taps and bone marrows.

When it [spinal taps and bone marrows] first started happening, it really hurt. I'd just lay on the table and screamed. But then like after a couple of times, I would just sit there and just let it happen because I was so like used to it. There was no use screaming because I had to go through with it until it is all over. So I would just calm down.

Joseph became quite knowledgeable about both his illness and his medications during his hospital stay.

I took it like a learning process in my life. The more I stayed [in the hospital] the more I learned. When I was about 8 [years old], I knew all the medications I was on. I knew what leukemia was . . . why I had it and what the problem was.

But his predominant memory of the time was that he just wanted to go home. "I wanted to be out of there [the hospital]. I wanted to go play with my friends and everything."

TREATMENT SIDE EFFECTS

Joseph had the common side effects associated with chemotherapy and radiation treatments. In the early stages of treatment, "I was all right. I was able to get up and push my IV around and pretty much go do things." Though hospitalized, he was not in isolation. "I was in a room with others. It wasn't like I had to be in intensive care or shut off from a certain group of people." The prednisone made him "real pudgy; you know it puffs your face out and stuff. It makes you gain weight." He lost his hair from the "tons of x-rays, plenty of radiation" that he experienced. Though Joseph suffered from nausea, vomiting, diarrhea, headaches, and fever, he claims that the side effects "really didn't bother me." Yet, midway through his treatment regime, there came a time when he felt so sick "I was totally out of it. I just couldn't do anything for myself. I couldn't eat, I couldn't do anything."

IMPACT ON THE FAMILY

Joseph's mother was unable to cope with his illness and its treatment regimes. As a result, just after he was diagnosed, he was assigned to a foster mother. He lived with her when he was not in the hospital, during the 4 years of his treatment protocol and beyond that time as well.

Medical records show that Joseph's natural mother visited him when he was hospitalized, and at times even spent the night in Joseph's room. The records also note that Joseph was anxious and nervous in the presence of his mother or when he thought that she was going to visit him. Joseph could understand the difficulties his mother faced in coping with his illness. "It brought her down just to see me down like that [so sick]." But after the illness, though his mother wanted him returned to her, Joseph opted to remain in foster care. And eventually, Joseph made the choice to terminate contact with her. "We don't associate anymore."

THE SCHOOL EXPERIENCE

Perhaps because Joseph spent so much time in the hospital, with his days structured and supervised, he managed to keep up with his schoolwork. The school sent a tutor and Joseph believes he worked "2–3 hours a day." "Sometimes when the teacher didn't have time, he would like send the work to me with what I had to do and how it had to be done." On those days "everyone would help me with that. So I didn't fall behind in any grades or anything."

Eventually, however, Joseph became too sick to concentrate on schoolwork. "I just became too sick to do anything." But by then "I didn't really want to do the schoolwork anyway. I wanted to *go* to school. But I couldn't."

When the time finally came for Joseph to leave the hospital and return to school, he had lost all of his hair. "I didn't really want to go to school with my hair like that. I felt like, wait until my hair grows back in, you know." But they wouldn't wait, and Joseph was afraid. It took lots of support from the medical staff to coax him back to school.

I was scared to leave. Because of all the friends I made and I had been there (hospital) so long. When you are young you get attached to something and [you] don't want to let go. But they like [said], "Go ahead, you can do it." [They said] like, "There is nothing to be afraid of."

"At first, I mean I felt like ashamed and embarrassed because you know I had no hair. I always kept a hat on." Then, a new school rule was introduced: "NO HATS!" and Joseph "could no longer hide. I was exposed." Joseph's classmates, ignorant about his illness, made fun of him and Joseph could not keep from fighting back. "Kids were making fun of me; I got into a lot of fights and trouble. It wasn't the side effects from the treatments that bothered me so much; it was other people's reaction to my side effects that bothered me."

In the beginning, Joseph kept his illness a secret. "I didn't want to tell anybody about [the illness] because it really bothered me at first. It really did bother me." Joseph wanted desperately to be accepted by his friends. He didn't want to be "different."

Joseph's teachers and the school nurse had been briefed by his foster mother before he returned to school, but he believes that "they were told not to inform any of the kids . . . not to bring it up." Then,

one day I was like forget it. Next time someone picks on me I am going to [tell] them what it is. And the first person I told was my one friend, Terrence. And him and me have been friends ever since. Then I told my girlfriend.

Once the secret was out, school became a very important part of Joseph's life, and of his recovery. School gave him "a second reason to want to keep on living."

School can make you feel like a normal kid again if it is handled in the right way. It can be a safe place to be during all the pain and chaos in your life. You don't feel like you are going to die if you are in school. It distracts your mind from what is happening to you.

Joseph's school absences were "about average." Although he frequently caught a cold, his oncologist "always had a remedy. And that's what made me want to do something in the medical field. Because I have always had people helping me, so I want to give back."

Joseph remembered being a straight A student in elementary school and junior high, although his grades did decline in high school. "[I got] straight As all the way until I got into high school because it got harder. Then I was like an A, B, C [student]. He also acknowledged with pride that his College Board score was "1100". Some of his school success Joseph attributes to his help from his friends. "I was offered lots of help especially by the girls. Like homework and stuff. Like the girls would constantly ask me. "Oh, can I help you?" after they found out [about me]. Joseph's teachers, on the other hand, did not give him any special help or preferential treatment. "They [the teachers] provided everybody with the same [treatment]. I remember one [teacher]. She told me she didn't want me feeling like I was isolated or singled out from the class, like I needed special attention. So, she treated everybody the same."

AREAS OF SCHOOL DIFFICULTY

Joseph reported no school learning problems whatsoever. "No reading problems. My comprehension is excellent. I loved math." He did acknowledge problems in concentrating, especially "when I first got out [of the hospital, I] would be looking at the board and seeing what the teacher was doing. I would just zone out and start thinking about other things."

Joseph believed that the tutoring he received while in the hospital helped his academic reintegration go smoothly because he knew what was going on in the class. He never felt as if he had fallen behind in any subject area.

That (tutoring) helped me a lot. So I mean, when I went back to school, I was right on time with the rest of the class. I knew what everybody was doing. I wasn't lost like how do you do this or how do you do that. I was just right along with the class. Everything they did, I knew about.

SURVIVING

Joseph believes that his cancer experience helped him grow up. As he puts it, "What kid wouldn't grow up fast from this experience? I was involved with adult issues like pain, loneliness, survival, and death. After what I went through, I consider myself grown." And he also carried around a feeling of shame for having been so sick. "I was ashamed to like tell people that I had leukemia." It has taken him a long time to put the illness in perspective, to put the illness behind him. He has accomplished that by reinterpreting his cancer experiences as "another of life's lessons" and trying to find the good that came out of those earlier times.

You know, something happens to you for a reason. [For] some people, the purpose is good. For some, it's not. And I feel my purpose was good. I think I got leukemia for a reason. God gave this disease to get me out of that bad neighborhood and to give me a second chance at becoming a good person. It was like God was talking to me, saying, "I don't want you to fall by the wayside because you got all these gangsters running around doing this, that, and the other. I'm [God] going to put you away for a little bit, [then] you are going to come back out, and you are going to be strong. You are going to be able to do things the right way." That is just the way I take it. He (God) did this to me for a reason. So I'm not going to sit here and say "Oh, I had leukemia now I can be a bum and go out using drugs, and this, that, and the other." I am going to make something out of myself.

Joseph is very optimistic about the future. He has put the cancer experience behind him. He does not feel compromised by it in any way.

I am over it! I'm all better! Now I am just like everybody else. Now I'm able to do anything and everything that I can possibly do. Anything that anyone else can do, I can go and do it. I can go play basketball. I can play football. I can swim. Ride a bike, ride a skateboard, drive a car. I can go hunting and fishing just like everybody else.

But he recognizes that the cancer experience shaped the way he approaches all challenges that come his way. "I really didn't let things get to me . . . I just did what I had to do. I am still that way . . . nothing really bothers me."

Joseph reported that the members of his family still worry about him, and are sensitive to and apprehensive about any change in his appearance or behavior.

Sometimes, there are days when I just don't feel good. I do not feel like doing anything. But I'm all right. I mean I know what it is. It is just like it is a bad day and everybody has them. But when I don't feel good, my sister will be like, "You should go to the doctor. You don't look too hot." I'm like, "I'm all right." You have bad days; you know what I'm saying. Ever since I turned 20, after work I would go out with my buddies, go to a club, or something. I'll come in at 4:00 a.m. and they [my family] will be like, "Where were you?" I tell them, "I am out having fun, that's all." They keep asking me and I know why they keep asking me. It's because they don't want anything to happen to me. Being sick has made them more protective of me.

Joseph does not worry that the cancer will return. "As far as I can see it, I have been in remission for about 8 years now. It is like long gone." But he is also unperturbed about the possibilities. "If it comes back up, then it comes back up. I will be able to deal with it a lot better than I did when I was younger. Because I already know what is expected of me."

During his years of illness and treatments, Joseph recalled two very positive influences that made his traumatic journey easier to accept and bear. One was the Make-A-Wish Foundation and the other was the American Cancer Society's Camp-Can-Do. These organizations provided him with wonderful memories and periods of escape from his ominous reality.

They [the Make-A-Wish Foundation] came and I forget where we went to buy things but we went shopping. I bought an arcade, radio, some tapes, and stuff like that. That was really nice. That was when I got out of the hospital for the first time. The American Cancer Society's [Camp-Can-Do]. Nothing but fun. Fun, fun, fun. It was a lot of fun. It was a massive escape from reality. Everybody there knew they had leukemia or some cancer but once you were there it was like it didn't matter. It was like you were you. There is nothing wrong. Nobody has anything. It was pretty cool.

Joseph feels that the cancer experience afforded him many opportunities for friendships. "I made a lot of friends along the way because of the type of person I am. I am an open person and can talk to people." It also changed him forever. "I do know it [the cancer experience] has made me a better man. Sure I feel different than my friends . . . I am different but in a better way. I am special." And it taught him some important life lessons.

It basically taught me about life. To me, I don't think there is nothing in this world worse than that [leukemia]. There is just nothing like [it]. I mean it is horrible. Then I made it through and I feel I made it through for a reason. I did this [the interview] because just like

I said, there is a purpose behind it. I've always wondered, "why did I make it? Why am I still here?" So I thought to myself to hold on. Maybe there is a purpose for my being left here. Maybe I can help somebody else that is going through the problem that I had. If I can help somebody else, I am willing to do it. After all, why are we all here if we don't reach out and help each other? More important, the dark shadows of that time have given me a light to guide me on my path in life today.

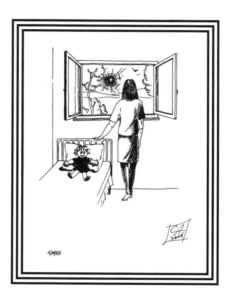

Dreams of a Future

10

Live in the Today and Dream of Tomorrow

Karen's Story

Today is a gift. Today I will let myself plan for the future
and live in the moment. I only have to live this day.
Nothing more is asked of me. I move courageously
in the directions of my dreams. I live in the now.

—Perry Tilleraas

Karen is a beautiful 18-year-old woman with flowing wavy medium-brown hair that lands just below her shoulders. She is 5'7". She lives with her parents and one brother, three years younger than she is.

Karen's cancer experience began in the spring of grade one, when she was 6 years old. The entire treatment regime lasted just over 2 years. She was treated with chemotherapy, but was never given radiation.

Karen is currently working part-time at the bakery of a local grocery store. She is planning to attend her first year of college in the fall. She will major in biology. She is "very excited!"

Karen seemed very comfortable talking about her illness experience, especially about her stays at Camp-Can-Do, which she considered "the best thing that happened to me." School was never a problem for Karen; her grades were above average even in the years when she missed a lot of school. But, although the battle with cancer does not seem to have left permanent psychological scars, Karen does look back on her childhood and concludes, "I really missed out on a lot of kid stuff at school."

ONSET OF THE DISEASE AND TREATMENT

During the early spring of first grade, Karen developed bruises around her knees and gradually, through the course of 1 week, had a number of bruises all over her body. "It wasn't because I was bumping into stuff. I was just getting them." One evening, at bedtime, Karen's mother noticed the large bruises on her feet and became alarmed. Her parents bundled her up and immediately took her to the local hospital.

I had black-and-blue marks all over the place, like some were on my arms (those were like little ones) and I had really huge black-and-blue marks on the top of my foot. That big one on my foot was what my mom looked at. I think she was putting me in the bath. It was really huge! My mom called my dad. Then they thought, "We better take her to the hospital."

Later that night, she was transferred to Children's Hospital. "I remember they took me by ambulance with the lights on! It was really exciting for me!"

When Karen was admitted to Children's Hospital of Pittsburgh, her medical records stated that she had thrombocytopenia (a blood condition in which the platelets in the blood are reduced, usually caused by a breakdown of tissue in the bone marrow), decreased white blood cells (cells that fight infection), hepatosplenomegaly (unusual enlargement of the spleen), and diffuse (widely spread) adenopathy (a growth or an enlargement of a lymph gland), all the symptoms common to acute leukemia. Karen was observed overnight and on the next day a bone marrow biopsy confirmed the diagnosis of childhood acute lymphoblastic leukemia. A spinal tap was also performed; it was negative for any leukemic cells in the CNS. Her parents were told on April 23, 1985, that Karen had ALL.

Karen was started immediately on the induction phase of chemotherapy, which consisted of vincristine (2.0 mg on days 0, 7, 14, 21, and 28), L-asparaginase (6,000U MWF, started on day 3), prednisone (40 mg on days 0–27 then taper over 14 days), and methotrexate IT (12 mg on days 0 and 14). Karen's induction phase was started on April 23, 1985, and lasted for 4 weeks. However, Karen was hospitalized for only 11 days. "It seemed like a long time but it was only 11 days." The rest of time she was given these medications on an outpatient basis. Karen tolerated the induction phase well, except for nausea and a urinary tract infection that was treated with bacterium therapy.

Karen's consolidation phase of chemotherapy treatment began on May 20, 1985, and ended on June 12, 1985, approximately 3 weeks. She received the chemotherapeutic agents of vincristine (1.5 mg on day 0), prednisone, 6-MP (75 mg on days 0–27), and methotrexate IT (12 mg on days 0, 7, 14, and 21).

Her maintenance phase of treatment began on June 18, 1985, and ended on May 30, 1987. Karen was in remission at the time and this phase lasted nearly 2 years. Her chemotherapy maintenance regime consisted of vincristine (monthly oral dose), 6-MP (daily), methotrexate (weekly oral dose), Methotrexate IT, and bone marrows and spinal taps. Her medical chart stated that Karen tolerated this stage of treatment very well.

By May 1987, the treatments were over and "ever since I got off the medication, I've been fine. I never went back for anything." She had experienced nausea, hair loss, and swelling, but no significant side effects and now, 9 years since her last chemotherapy treatment, there has been no recurrence of leukemia or any secondary forms of cancer.

KAREN'S REACTIONS TO DIAGNOSIS AND TREATMENT

When Karen thought back to her illness and treatments, the word that came to mind to describe the survival journey was *exciting*. Karen got to know the nurses and doctors really well, and this personal contact sustained her.

I knew all the nurses and doctors really good. I knew them by name when I'd go back for visits. It was exciting. That was really important to me. It didn't bother me as much when they would come in and take blood, you know, because it would be like, "Oh, it's Nurse Judy!"

Karen's outpatient visits for medication or tests "became routine. I'd like go and play there." For moral support, Karen relied heavily on a Cabbage Patch doll that shared her every experience. "When I was in the hospital, I had a Cabbage Patch doll with me. And everything I got, it got too. There are still Band-Aid marks on its arm [from the IV]. I mean that doll went with me everywhere."

Karen took her chemotherapy treatments in stride. For example, "I got to know the shots. There was one shot I'd get in my leg and I'd be like, 'This doesn't even hurt me. I didn't feel it or anything.'" But then, there were the spinal taps ("I did *not* like those!") and the bone marrow biopsies ("That was worse than the spinal taps!").

TREATMENT SIDE EFFECTS

Karen experienced the side effects common to the drugs in her protocol. She remembers being "very weak and skinny. I'd sleep a lot. I had very little energy. I missed out on things because I was so tired all the time." She also remembers that her "face was real puffy from the medicine." But the most difficult side effect was losing her hair. "I remember having no hair when I went back to school in the second grade. I was almost totally bald." After losing her hair, the texture of the new hair growth changed dramatically. [Before I lost my hair], it was straight and blond. It was really long! It came back in brown and wavy. I thought, "Oh God, I hate this!"

Despite the changes she experienced, Karen never considered her physical appearance to be a big issue, probably because she was so young at the time. However, Karen did acknowledge that if she had been older, the impact would have been greater.

I don't know how I dealt with that (physical appearance). I know if I had been older, it would have been a much bigger issue. I would have been more worried about the peer pressure, "What do these people think of me?" But in second grade, I was pretty much there to have fun!

Karen never talked much about her feelings during this time. Reflecting back on it now, she believes that the illness caused her to miss out on important life activities. For example, during the birthday party celebrating age 7,

It was my party and everyone was playing softball. Maybe it was right after I was diagnosed? I remember we had this huge field next to our house and everybody was playing softball. I felt really left out because I couldn't play. I just had no energy. It was like my whole family [was] playing and I'd walk back up to the house alone and lay down. I remember waking up to open up my presents and then I'd go back to sleep. I was really tired all the time. So that's when I just started keeping things to myself . . . not even disclosing my feelings to my family. I never said anything about that day . . . how I felt about it. But I always felt left out.

IMPACT ON THE FAMILY

Karen remembers her family as having been "really protective of me . . . really protective."

I think at first my parents just didn't want me to hurt more than I had to because of the leukemia. Parents feel a sense of helplessness when they see their child suffering. Then they end up being even more protective so nothing else happens to that child.

Karen's baby brother, only 3 years old at the time of her diagnosis, "was just running around in diapers. I think maybe if my brother had been older, he would have been a lot more affected by the attention that I got and he didn't get." As it was, he seemed oblivious to Karen's crises.

Karen spoke very little about her parents' reactions to her illness. She had very little to say about her family's reactions at the time of her illness and treatments or even today.

THE SCHOOL EXPERIENCE

Karen has always viewed school as important but she never felt her parents pushed her to do well in school. They didn't have to; she pushed herself. "School wasn't usually hard for me. I've always been on the honor roll and that's just myself pushing me along. My parents really . . . they have said, 'Go to college,' and this and that, but it was me pushing myself along."

Karen was in first grade when she was diagnosed with ALL; it was April, and she started treatments immediately. She was tutored for the remainder of her first-grade year. "I would think that my mother talked to the tutor about me. I don't remember much about it."

At the beginning of second grade, Karen returned to school. Karen said that it was her mother who communicated with her teachers but both her mother and father worked with her at home on worksheets during her illness. She shared,

I'm sure my mom did [spoke to the teachers]. Not my dad. But that was before the tutoring. My parents . . . I remember in first, second, and third grades . . . always sitting down and helping me with the spelling back in the early years. [They] always sat down and helped me. My mom and dad would go over worksheets with me and stuff like that.

She wished that her mom and dad would have had more interested in her education.

I don't think my parents have ever been really active in my education. Like my younger brother, he struggles through school. Like he always used to be average. But he just really

isn't studying and that's not his thing. I've always pushed myself. I always want to do good. Not even to impress my parents, but to impress myself. I've always done that so I do sorta wish they would've been more interested.

Karen remembered that she would go home excited about her report card and wanting her parents' attention, approval, and pride about her schoolwork.

I would always run up to [them] on report card day . . . they might not even know it was report card day. Then I'd be like, "Look what I did!" I did really good. I was so proud of myself. I've always been like that.

Karen was reintegrated into school at the start of second grade. Perhaps that is why she felt the closest to her second-grade teacher.

My second-grade teacher . . . she was really nice. I was really close to her. I think she gave me special attention. I'm sure she went around and helped everybody, but she was really nice to me. Especially with my school[work] . . . with stuff I could not grasp or comprehend. It really isn't anything that sticks out in my mind, but I remember that she was always really, really nice to me. [She was] the only teacher who [made me feel] special. I don't know what she knew about me. . . . I think she was informed what I had been through. But that is the teacher I remember the most.

A special bond developed between Karen and this teacher. Karen recalled that "right after second grade we moved to West Mifflin [a suburb of Pittsburgh]. I just kept thinking, I've got to call my teacher. I've got to talk to my teacher! Because I was really, really close to her."

Changing schools was hard for Karen. This second-grade teacher had helped her over a big hurdle. "In second grade I had like no hair at the beginning of the year. I was bald." To ease the transition, Karen's mother arranged for her to take home some crayons that had been distributed in class.

My mom took me to class. They [the other second graders] were all there. We were never allowed to take our crayons home. I don't really remember any of the kids that I was friends with back then, but I remember everybody looking at me saying, "She gets to take her crayons home." Then I said good-bye to my teacher and we left.

The transition to third grade in the new school was difficult. Karen was still taking the treatments for cancer. As far as she could tell, her mother did not tell anyone at her new school about her health. Third grade became her most difficult school year. She expressed her thoughts and feelings about that school year.

When I went into third grade, I don't think my mom had said anything to the teacher. I don't think anyone in the school really knew about me at first. Third grade was really hard for me. To like pick up, move, meet all these new people, and still be having cancer treatments was a lot for me to deal with at the time. Schooling-wise, that was my hardest year. It was just such a big change. I think I was a little bit scared to meet new people. If somebody would say something to me about being sick. . . . I still sometimes don't know how to react to . . . what they say or whatever. But there was so much different stuff going on and schooling got really hard for me.

Despite these difficulties, Karen soon made friends. "I mean I had a lot of friends. I'm still friends with them now. My best friend in the third grade is one of my best friends now." And teachers tried to give her special tasks to help her feel important and needed. For example, in the third grade, "I use[d] to check papers for the teacher like spelling quizzes," and in fifth grade, "I'd fill in for the secretary during her lunch hour."

Karen does not remember telling anyone the truth about her illness until the sixth grade. Throughout those early years of school, Karen struggled with a need to share her experiences and a strong desire not to have people think she was different because of having had cancer as a child. Karen thought that telling people about her cancer might be inappropriate.

When I'd go to school after being out [absent because of treatments or side effects of treatments], . . . like I didn't want to say anything. I didn't want them to think I was weird, I was different.

At Camp-Can-Do, I could say anything there. But at school, it was like don't say anything. If somebody mentioned leukemia . . . [I kept wondering] should I say anything. [But] I didn't because I didn't want to start anything. Like I remember one time in health class, I felt like saying, "I went through this. I know what this is and I know what that is and I can describe this for you." But I didn't want to go there.

And, Karen believes, because of the cancer treatments she missed out on a lot of important childhood experiences.

Like when the other kids were doing this and that I was losing my hair and I was weak. I was really tired all the time from all my medicine. I was taking like ten pills a day. I couldn't be in sports and clubs and stuff like that. I feel like I REALLY missed out on that kind of kid stuff. Then later on it was hard to say, "Well I'm going to start this sport now" when all these kids had all this experience. I really regret it.

Then, in sixth grade, a history teacher "a really mean history teacher . . . like he should have been an advanced teacher . . . teaching an older group of [kids] assigned the class an essay to write."

That was the first time that I had ever written that I had gone through ALL as a child . . . cancer. I remember he pulled me aside afterward like after he read the papers. He said, "Did you really go through this?" Then he said, "I have great admiration for you." Then it like really hit me because I had never said anything to any of my teachers before about going through what I did. When I told that teacher, I felt really good. Like . . . I felt like I had been through something rougher than the rest of these kids.

Looking back on those years, Karen felt that school "was an anchor for me."

. . . something in my life that was forced to continue in spite of what was happening around me. Sometimes it made feel like I was just like the rest of the kids. . . . I think going to school was a good effort in trying make me feel like everything was "normal" when it was far from being "normal."

AREAS OF SCHOOL DIFFICULTY

What Karen remembered was that "school wasn't hard for me. I've always been on the honor roll and that's just myself pushing me along. My parents really . . . they said this and that, but it was me pushing myself along." Karen's best academic subject was reading; she was always "in advanced reading." But math was hard for her.

I'm not real good at math! I remember forever trying to learn the multiplication facts. I hated it! My homeroom teacher was a math teacher. He loved math! He wore ties and math shirts that had numbers all over the place! It was horrible! It was the memorization of those facts. I just couldn't do it. Then later on I had a lot of trouble with algebra and geometry.

Karen recalled being absent from school frequently. After being diagnosed with cancer in April of first grade, she was tutored at home for the remainder of the school year. In second grade, she had numerous absences due to doctor's appointments and being sick from the treatments.

I know I had really bad attendance from doctor's appointments and being sick from the drugs and all in second grade. I missed out on a lot in school both academically and socially. Sometimes you can't play catch up when it deals with losing time.

But Karen was never retained. The tutoring she received kept her from having to be "held back."

SURVIVING

Karen went to work at a beauty salon when she was 15 because her mother had worked there too. The receptionist at the salon turned out to have been Karen's school nurse from elementary school. Karen did not recognize her but this retired school nurse certainly remembered Karen. She told Karen a very positive story about how Karen's illness had helped this woman when another student in the school was diagnosed with cancer.

She told me that she knew what leukemia was all about because of me. It was really helpful for her . . . her being informed about me and having to know all about my medicines and illness. She said knowing me helped her with that person. I think that was the first time that I realized something good came from having cancer as a kid.

One of the most significant experiences contributing to her physical, psychological, emotional, and social adjustment was a camp that children with cancer can participate in once a year, Camp-Can-Do, sponsored by the American Cancer Society. Her memories and reminiscences are extremely positive. It was a place for her to "let go" and "regroup" since she could not do that in other parts in her life.

Every year up until 2 years ago, I always went to a Camp-Can-Do... everybody there has been diagnosed with some kind of cancer. Whether they were in remission or not, those were like my closest friends I've ever had. Every year you go back and that was really, really helpful. People who were going through the same things as me. It was really helpful to help other people after I had already made it to remission . . . like talking to them . . . what I went through . . . Really, in the schools, you know, I couldn't talk there but at this camp you could talk to the people there about anything. It was like okay. Any questions . . . what you were going through? I'm going through this. How do you feel about this?

Karen hopes to go back to this camp as a counselor herself when she is 20. She believes that since she survived acute leukemia that she could give hope to children who are battling the same disease.

It was really great when I was little and I knew these older kids and they came back. Then I'd show up one year as a camper and they were a counselor! I thought, "You went through this! You were once a camper!" I just thought that was great! I am definitely going to do that! That was really . . . the best thing . . . talking to someone who had been through it.

Camp-Can-Do provided Karen with a second family and a place where she could just be herself. It was a safe and secure environment for her during a very troubling and painful time.

That (Camp-Can-Do) was one of the best things that ever happened to me! I talked to one of my counselors today. I'm really close to her. She just called me today. As soon as I heard her voice, I was so happy! I mean, it's just I feel so secure with those people. They were like my second family. I got like closer to them than probably my friends at home. So that (camp) was the best thing that came out of everything.

From time to time, Karen wonders why she survived when so many children do not make it.

It just drives me crazy. I don't have an answer for myself, let alone trying to tell someone else why I think I survived this disease. It would be nice in a way if God came down and said I spared your life because of this or that. On the other hand, then you would have to live up to great expectations and what if you didn't measure up, then what?

However, she does not dwell on that. Instead, she concentrates on making the "right decisions" about her future. She feels a strong need to give back to other children who are experiencing cancer.

I don't really think every day, "I'm going to cherish this day because of what I went through." I don't think like that. But I do know and believe that I am very different from other people because of experiencing leukemia as a child. It certainly builds character and it makes you look at things very differently. Yeah, I think I am special for having survived this, and I feel any kid who survives leukemia is special. It's really, really important that I go back as a counselor [to Camp-Can-Do] and help younger kids go through everything that I went through.

The experience of having childhood cancer has made Karen live in the today and not dwell on the past.

I don't go through every single day thinking about what happened to me. But there are days when I just can't shake the impact it has had on me, and I think I better cherish this day because of what I experienced as a child. . . . I'm trying really, really hard to just live in the today of my life and yet dream about my tomorrows. I'm actually thinking about my dreams now, trying hard to leave the past behind me. I never thought I would be saying this to someone but it does make me feel really good to say to you, "I am starting to plan a future . . . my future."

Part II

Surviving Survival

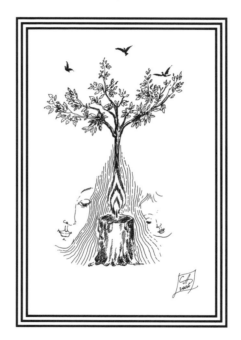

From Childhood to Adulthood! The Light of Hope

11

Physiological, Psychological, and Social Side Effects

Solving Some Problems and Creating New Ones

PHYSIOLOGICAL SIDE EFFECTS

> Cancer is an unsettling reminder of the obdurate grain of unpredictability and uncertainty and injustice—value questions all in the human condition. Cancer points up our failure to explain and confront our lack of control. Perhaps most fundamentally, cancer symbolizes our need to make moral sense of "why me?" that scientific explanations cannot provide. Cancer is also freighted with the risks . . . of anticancer drugs as poisons . . . and implicate[s] medical technology as part of the danger.
>
> —Arthur Kleinman, *The Illness Narratives*

Childhood cancer is slowly being eradicated. But as the nine stories illustrate, traveling the road to cure takes courage and stamina, and the battle leaves lasting scars. Each journey to survival is unique; each child in each family uniquely struggles through the cancer experience. Nevertheless, even in this small sample of stories, we see common patterns, common threads. Understanding these commonalties and being informed may help others anticipate them, plan for them, or at least accept them as "normal" obstacles on the road to cure and may even improve their eventual outcome.

Transient Physiological Side Effects

The biomedical research literature is replete with reports of the physiological side effects of antileukemic therapy. Chemotherapy and radiation inevitably produce transient (temporary) as well as long-term side effects as they bombard both abnormal and normal body tissue. Nausea and vomiting, fluid retention, weight gain, hair loss, fever, and diarrhea have all been reported in the research literature (see, for example, Tyc, Mulhern, & Bieberich, 1997) and were also reported by the survivors whose stories are told in this book. Physiological side effects that can be both transient and long term that may impact survivors are chronic pain, loss of energy, muscle weakness, loss of sensation/partial paralysis, fatigue, sleep problems, behavior problems, mental confusion, irritability, anemia, visual impairment, muscle aches, and mouth sores (Spinelli, 2003). Those children who are fighting the disease or are long-term survivors may also have compromised immunity systems that can promote an increase in infections and viruses (Spinelli, 2003). Survivors also learned to live with migraine headaches, sterility or infertility, stunted growth, and poor resistance to infections (National Cancer Institute, 2002). Their accounts of these side effects remind us that, although the physical symptoms may pass quickly, the psychological repercussions may last considerably longer. As Timothy put it, "It doesn't make you an outcast because you have it [cancer]. It makes you feel like an outcast because of the side effects, like losing your hair or swelling. It makes you feel like you're not the same as everybody else."

As Table 11.1 shows, the nine respondents suffered from a variety of side effects. One side effect is that the cells of the stomach and the intestine are also ferociously attacked by the toxic chemotherapy used to treat cancer. The result is sometimes vomiting, sometimes diarrhea, or both. Six of the nine respondents reported nausea and vomiting associated with their chemotherapy treatments and spinal taps. Elaine, Ruth, and Joseph shared issues related to diarrhea.

All nine respondents were on prednisone at one time or another during the course of their treatment regimes, and all reported experiencing the most common side effect of prednisone, weight gain and swelling or puffiness. All nine respondents experienced high fevers at various junctures of their treatment protocols. For some, the fevers were associated with chicken pox, for others, with pneumonia, and for still others, with infections. However, in all cases, the fevers dissipated after the end of the medical crisis.

Chemotherapy drugs destroy not only cancer cells that are produced at a rapid rate, but also normal cells. Because hair follicle cells reproduce quickly, chemotherapy causes some or all body hair to fall out. The hair on the scalp,

TABLE 11.1
Transient Physiological Side Effects

Symptoms	Reported by
Nausea and Vomiting	Frank, Patricia, Timothy, Matthew, Lynn, Karen
Fluid Retention/Weight Gain	Frank, Patricia, Elaine, Timothy, Matthew, Lynn, Ruth, Joseph, Karen
Fever	Frank, Patricia, Elaine, Timothy Matthew, Lynn, Ruth, Joseph, Karen
Hair Loss	Frank, Patricia, Elaine, Timothy, Matthew, Lynn, Ruth, Joseph, Karen
Diarrhea	Elaine, Ruth, Joseph
Headaches	Patricia, Lynn
Infectious Diseases	Frank, Patricia, Elaine, Lynn, Ruth
Pneumonia	Patricia, Elaine, Ruth

eyebrows, eyelashes, underarms, and pubic area may slowly thin out or may fall out in big clumps. Hair growth usually reoccurs 1 to 3 months after maintenance starts or intensive chemotherapy ends. The color and texture of the hair may change when it begins to grow back. All nine respondents reported hair loss. In addition, Patricia and Lynn reported struggling with headaches associated with the cancer treatments and spinal taps.

With a compromised immune system, children undergoing cancer treatments are very susceptible to infectious diseases. Five of the survivors reported bouts of chicken pox, measles, or mononucleosis. Chicken pox can be a very serious, even life-threatening, disease for a child who has leukemia, both during and after treatments. Measles is an acute, highly contagious viral disease that occurs foremost in children. Mononucleosis is an abnormal increase in the number of mononuclear white blood cells in circulation; its symptoms are very close to those of leukemia. Patricia, Elaine, and Ruth also suffered bouts of pneumonia.

Long-Term Physiological Side Effects

Although most of the side effects of the disease and of the treatments received to combat the disease were short term and transient, some left long-term scars, both literally and figuratively. Table 11.2 shows the long-term physiological side effects experienced by seven of the nine respondents.

TABLE 11.2
Long-Term Physiological Side Effects

Symptom	Reported by
Gonadal and Endocrine Dysfunction	Patricia, Timothy, Matthew, Ruth
Skin Problems	Elaine, Timothy, Matthew, Ruth
Problems with Bones and Teeth	Timothy, Matthew, Lynn, Ruth
Poor Resistance to Infections	Patricia, Ruth
Migraine Headaches	Frank, Patricia, Timothy, Elaine
Relapse or Secondary Cancers	Patricia, Ruth

The literature is abound with reports of sterility and testicular atrophy in boys as a consequence of radiation or chemotherapy. In this set of stories, two of the four males, Matthew and Timothy, reported testicular atrophy. Matthew assumed that he was sterile and his doctor assumed so as well. Timothy, on the other hand, did not accept this assumption and "tested it out." He is the happy father of two children.

In early reports of long-term consequences of cancer treatment, the majority of girls did not seem to suffer from infertility or ovarian dysfunction. Elaine reported that she had regular menstrual periods and hoped that she would be able to one day have a baby. But more recently, Marina (1997) found that some females do experience premature menopause and infertility from chemotherapy. This happened to be the case with both Ruth and Patricia.

Skin problems are a common side effect of cancer treatments. Timothy and Matthew both reported difficulty in growing facial hair such as a mustache or beard. Elaine and Ruth were both troubled by scars left on their bodies as physical reminders of the experience. Elaine's were primarily the result of her cancer treatments, though the final blow was from gallbladder surgery. She felt from her perspective that there was not one place on her body that was not scarred by the cancer experience. Ruth developed scars from facial shingles associated with her bone marrow transplants. Both women worried that the scars would permanently affect their physical appearance.

Several investigators have reported significant stunted growth in both boys and girls as a result of chemotherapy or radiation treatments for cancer. In these stories, one boy and two girls had this side effect from their cancer treatments. Matthew thought he would have been 2 to 3 inches taller if he had not had the disease and the treatments, since all of the members of his immediate family are at least 3 to 4 inches taller than his current height. Lynn's medical records indicate that she should have been 3 to 4 inches taller than her current height of 4'11". Ruth's medical records also note an effect on her height but the records did not indicate by what degree her height was affected by the cancer experience. Ruth was 5 feet tall as an adult.

Another permanent side effect seen in the sample in this book was brittle teeth (reported by Timothy) or brittle bones (reported by Ruth). In Matthew's and Lynn's medical records, there was mention of issues with their teeth. Research tells us that the younger the age of diagnosis the more likely it is that radiation administered to the head area can cause poor tooth enamel, root formation, gum disease, and brittle teeth (Marina, 1997).

For two respondents, Patricia and Ruth, poor resistance to infections followed them from the time of their cancer treatments right into adulthood. Extensive chemotherapy treatments over a few years may cause a compromised immunity system over the long term. Frank, Elaine, Timothy, and Patricia all suffer today with chronic migraine headaches. Cancer treatment of intrathecal methotrexate and radiation to the head area is known to cause the long-term side effect of migraine headaches.

Two of the nine survivors (Patricia and Ruth) fought cancer a second time years after they were in remission from ALL as young children. According to Marina (1997) such occurrences are not rare. Researchers estimate that 3–12% of children treated for childhood cancer will develop a secondary form of cancer (most likely leukemia or solid tumors) within 20 years of diagnosis, with the risk of secondary leukemia reaching a plateau at 10–15 years from diagnosis.

PSYCHOLOGICAL AND SOCIAL CHALLENGES

> By their full, active, and hopeful lives . . . children living with cancer [and surviving cancer] are teaching us all how to live.
>
> —John J. Spinetta

The diagnosis and treatment of childhood cancer is an extremely stressful and traumatic experience. The chronic strains of childhood cancer—such as treatment-related pain; nausea and vomiting; visible side effects of hair loss, weight gain/loss, and physical disfigurement; and repeated absences from school and peers—must certainly have an impact on the developing child. Most childhood cancer survivors do not have long-term, clinically significant psychological difficulties; most function well as children and into their adult lives (Kazak, 1994). But to the young child, the battle with cancer is especially hard and scary; its psychological consequences can persist many years after the end of treatment (Stuber et al., 1997).

The survivors spoke openly of their psychological traumas, but they also spoke of the methods they used to cope and to adjust to the stresses and strains of the cancer experience. The storytellers talked about how childhood cancer left them with an abbreviated childhood, which in turn caused accelerated maturity, never fitting in with their peer group, cancer paranoia, and survivor's guilt. Table 11.3 summarizes some common psychological and social challenges experienced by the respondents and the ways in which the cancer experience impacted their psychological and social development.

Surviving cancer means learning to tolerate painful medical procedures like spinal taps, bone marrow biopsies aspirations, needles, and so on, and, according to the respondents, "You never get used to it." Every one of the respondents discussed how painful the medical procedures

TABLE 11.3
Psychological and Social Challenges

Challenge	Reported by
Tolerating Chemotherapy and Painful Medical Procedures	Frank, Elaine, Timothy, Matthew
Learning the Truth about the Illness	Frank, Patricia, Elaine, Timothy, Matthew, Lynn
Dealing with Medical Personnel	Frank, Patricia, Elaine, Timothy, Matthew, Lynn, Ruth, Joseph, Karen
Feeling Different from Others	Patricia, Elaine, Lynn, Ruth, Joseph, Karen
Survivor Guilt	Elaine, Matthew, Lynn, Joseph, Karen
Growing Up Quickly	Patricia, Elaine, Ruth, Joseph, Karen
Optimistic Personality/ Positive Attitude	Frank, Elaine, Timothy, Ruth, Karen
Sense of Spirituality/ Sense of Purpose	Frank, Patricia, Elaine, Timothy, Matthew, Lynn, Ruth, Joseph, Karen

had been for them. Ruth and Frank remembered how awful the drugs made them feel. Patricia had vivid memories of the spinal taps. But Timothy thought that the bone marrow biopsies were the worst. For each of these survivors, their memories were vivid even though they had been very young at the time. These experiences left an indelible imprint in their minds that time could not erase.

The survivors also remembered how hard it was to learn the truth about their illness. How do parents tell their 5- or 6-year-old that she or he has cancer? What words do parents use to explain the illness to their child, when they do not understand it themselves? The answer is that many do not talk about the cancer; some do not talk about the illness at all. Lynn always thought that she had a very bad cold or the flu. Timothy assumed he had pneumonia. Patricia remembers being told that she was sick because she had pneumonia and measles at the same time.

Whether they are told, explicitly or not, many children can deduce the seriousness of their illness from observing the people and events in their surroundings. For example, Matthew could not understand why he was so sick but he recognized that it was serious. Elaine, too, reported knowing that she was a very sick little girl. Frank figured it out when a hospital friend died from leukemia. For several of the survivors, the truth of their illness was not disclosed until some years after they had been in remission. It wasn't until he was 15 that Timothy found out the truth, and the memory of that afternoon of disclosure is still very vivid. Patricia was finally told at age 17 that she had had leukemia when she was 6 years old and she was shocked at the disclosure. She was very upset with her family for not telling her the truth sooner. In contrast, Matthew seemed grateful that his parents waited to tell him the particulars of his disease. Matthew's parents also kept it a secret from anyone outside of the immediate family and a few very close friends. Matthew thought that this had been a good decision for him.

All nine respondents remarked about the relationships they developed with medical personnel during the course of their illness. These relationships, whether positive or negative, impacted strongly on the memories of the cancer experience that the survivors carried with them through adolescence and into adulthood.Frank remembered a very difficult set of interactions early in his illness with a female physician whom he did not like; these negative feelings created turbulence in Frank's relationship with his mother because he blamed her for his assignment to this "bad" doctor. Elaine and Patricia also reported some negative experiences with a particular technician or a particular nurse.

But even these survivors also had wonderful memories of supportive and caring doctors and nurses. Elaine told stories of one nurse and one doctor who were particularly good to her. For Frank and Karen, having a positive personal relationship with the doctors and nurses helped them get through this painful and fearful experience. Timothy and Matthew came to think of the doctors and nurses as another family. Patricia and Ruth both thought they had "terrific" doctors, and Joseph not only liked his doctor, but also, trusted him completely.

Chesler, Weigers, and Lawther (1992) report that some cancer survivors see their survival as a victory. These young people may feel they have engaged in, and mastered a test, qualifying them for "special status." Even while the young people I interviewed acknowledged their physical and emotional scars, they often sounded and felt like victors rather than victims. All of the women and one of the men felt they had been changed, significantly, by the survival experience. They had a sense of accomplishment and of "specialness."

But several of them also suffered from survivor guilt; they were plagued by the question of why they survived when so many other individuals did not make it. For Elaine, Matthew, Lynn, Joseph, and Karen, surviving did not always promote a positive outlook, a sense of having beaten the odds, of having been victorious in a life-threatening battle. For them, surviving also had the opposite effect; they felt guilty instead of triumphant, and searched for an answer to the question, "Why me instead of someone else?" This survivor guilt became an added psychological and emotional burden. A few of the respondents commented while telling their stories that perhaps it was time to seek out some help in dealing with their cancer experience even though it was so many years later.

Fighting cancer takes a lot of energy, both physical and psychological, and, indeed, five of the nine storytellers believed that childhood cancer had caused them to lose out on many childhood experiences and to mature very quickly. Patricia, Ruth, and especially Karen felt cheated. Elaine and Joseph recognized their missed childhood opportunities but believed that, despite the trauma, they came out of it pretty well.

Most of the respondents in this book projected personalities that were upbeat, spunky, optimistic, positive, and bubbly. One wonders whether this optimistic personality and positive attitude was the very reason they survived the cancer experience.

God and a sense of spirituality certainly surfaced as a common theme within these interviews. Sometimes, the spirituality was reflected in statements like "God saved me for a reason," "God was looking out for me," or "I thank God that I am still here." Frank spoke about his spirituality in simple terms and with straightforwardness. Timothy was surprisingly direct in thanking God for keeping him here. Lynn and her mother and Patricia and her dad believed that a "divine power" intervened to save Lynn's and Patricia's life. Matthew and Ruth believed that their illness was something God had handed them and they had to simply handle it. They felt there was no alternative to their predicament but God was present and constantly watching them going through the experience. Ruth wondered what purpose God had for her now. Joseph trusted that his bout with cancer was part of God's bigger plan for him.

Eight of the nine respondents felt a strong need to give back to others in some way, to make their saved lives meaningful and purposeful. This is not an unusual reaction to surviving. According to Chesler et al. (1992), many adult long-term survivors look for opportunities to share their experiences and help others. Some write books about their experiences with cancer (for example, Gilda Radner, Jill Ireland, Betty Rollins). Others get involved in fund-raising, starting a support group, working for a cancer organization, donating money for research or for other expenses, or volunteering their time to organizations or foundations. The respondents in this book had the same innate instincts. Lynn and Frank keep looking for ways to give back. Frank and Timothy makes a point of helping other children who have cancer when he is getting an annual checkup at his doctor's office. Elaine believes that she became a pediatric nurse in order to help other children get through their illnesses. She also works with the Make-A-Wish Foundation. Patricia contributed money to Children's Hospital through a fund-raiser that her sister participated in because of Patricia's cancer experience. Lynn was in college to become a teacher; she believed that God helped her survive so that one day she could help other children. Ruth also dreams of helping sick children and their families, as well as raising money for cancer research. Ruth shared that if she were rich she would "like to have a ranch and have a weekend thing for these kids who are sick because all they see are hospitals. Get them out and take like five families and stay at the ranch and be able to ride horses and just have one hell of a ball for a weekend and just forget about everything. It would be free of charge. And if they wanted to pay anything, it would go toward [cancer] research." Joseph was heading off to college to pursue a career as a physical therapist "because of everything that happened to me." He also would like to be a counselor one day at the American Cancer Society's Camp-Can-Do. Karen also felt an intense bond with Camp-Can-Do and their counselors and hoped some day to go back to the camp as a counselor.

IMMEDIATE- AND LONG-TERM STRESS IN THE FAMILY
AND IN OTHER PERSONAL RELATIONSHIPS

Cancer strikes the entire family.

—Doris Lund

Learning to live with cancer is clearly no easy task. Learning
to live with someone else's cancer may be even more difficult,
precisely because no one recognizes just how hard it really is.

—Marilyn T. Oberst

Denial may serve as a useful method to survive the first days
after diagnosis, but a gradual acceptance must occur so that
the family can begin to make the necessary adjustments to
cancer treatment. Life has dramatically changed.

—Nancy Keene

When one member of a family has cancer, everything in that family changes. In an article in the *Pittsburgh Post-Gazette*, Srikameswaran (1994) stated how absolutely "profound the impact" is on the individual diagnosed with cancer and that individual's family.

In the process of coping with cancer, lives are permanently changed. Nobody who is diagnosed with cancer ever goes back. . . . When there's a cancer in the family, everything comes out of the woodwork. When it's one person [in the family with cancer], he [or she] becomes the center of the family and that's where all the energy can be focused, getting that person to treatment, helping them manage the side effects. It may be difficult to find the time to absorb the shock simply because there is too much to be done. People [in the family] often have to reorder their priorities. Initially, the cancer does rule your life and it's very big. Then people just learn it will always be a part of their lives. It's a different kind of normal. (pp.1, 15–16)

In the process of coping with cancer, the lives of all members of the family unit are permanently changed. Some parents adjust well to the sudden change in their lives, and they fulfill their usual daily tasks quite adequately (Hoekstra-Weebers, Jaspers, Kamps, & Klip, 1998). More commonly, however, parents experience intense psychological distress, anxiety, and depression (Hoekstra-Weebers et al., 1998). According to Keene (1999), not only the individual is mourning the loss of their past life but parents undergo a grieving process in which they are mourning the loss of a life of normalcy and knowing life will never be the same. Many parents become physically ill for weeks after their child is newly diagnosed, from not eating properly, not getting enough sleep, exposure to illness in the hospital, and excruciating emotional stress. Some parents experience a dreamlike state similar to shock in which the brain provides protective layers of numbness and confusion to prevent emotional overload (Keene, 1999). After a time, the physical symptoms may fade, but the intense emotional effects continue for quite some time. Interestingly, childhood cancer survivors and their families have been known to use denial as a coping strategy to such a life-altering, life-threatening trauma (Phipps, Fairclough, & Mulhern, 1995).

Fathers and mothers may react quite differently to the diagnosis of their child having cancer. Hoekstra-Weebers et al. (1998) found "a shift took place from distress in fathers, shortly after diagnosis, to more distress in mothers 12 months later" (p. 26). They believed this was due to roles set forth within the family. According to Hoekstra-Weebers et al. (1998), fathers after 12 months go back to their usual life of going to work on a regular basis but mothers still have the major burden of taking care of the child, whether they have a job or not. It was a shared responsibility for both mothers and fathers at diagnosis but 12 months later mothers may feel deserted because they are still handling the child's doctor's appointments, treatments, side effects, and emotional difficulties. Mothers also expressed higher stress levels because it was usually their role to deal with the child's issues in school both academically and socially after diagnosis and during treatments.

Fathers are more likely to blame doctors for failing to diagnose the condition; mothers search for causes closer to home and are less likely to accept that there is no known cause for the child's illness (Eiser, Havermans, & Eiser, 1995). After the initial diagnosis and treatments, fathers often become engrossed in their work, feeling that if they are working, they are doing their part in helping with the child's care. Mothers may grow resentful as they assume more and more responsibility for their sick child's care. Many mothers of children with leukemia turn to tranquilizers, antidepressants, or sleeping pills to get through their days and nights.

Some family units grow more cohesive, pull together in the time of crisis (Rait et al., 1992). For others, the illness of one family member can lead to dysfunction and discord, leaving family members feeling disconnected and unsupported (Rait et al., 1992). To avoid long-term difficulties, support services are often recommended to assist with family communication and the development of effective coping strategies. Unfortunately, psychological adjustment may be determined by uncontrollable factors such as absence of learning difficulties, absence of functional and physical limitations, and not coming from a single-parent home (Kazak, 1994).

> A diagnosis of leukemia strips parents of control over their child's daily life. Previously, parents established routines and rules which defined family life. Children woke up, washed and dressed, ate breakfast, perhaps attended day care or school, played with friends, and performed chores. Life was predictable. Suddenly, the family is thrust into a new world populated by an everchanging cast of characters (interns, residents, fellows, oncologists, IV teams, nurses, social workers), and containing new language (medical terminology: a new world full of hospitalizations, procedures, and drugs).
>
> —Nancy Keene, *Childhood Leukemia: A Guide for Families, Friends, and Caregivers*

The families of survivors in this book experienced many of the stresses and strains reported in the research literature. The survivors described the reactions of both mothers and fathers to their diagnoses and to the ongoing treatment regimes. They described stresses in their parents' marriages exacerbated by the cancer and the financial burdens that treatments produced. And they described immediate and long-lasting difficulties with siblings that they attributed to the childhood cancer experience. (See Table 11.4.)

Eiser et al. (1995) conducted a study about the affects on mothers versus fathers once the child has been diagnosed with cancer. The mothers become more emotional, religious, confident, loving, and sensitive. The fathers become more aware of disabilities, maturer in values, and more aggressive. Another study done by Dahlquist, Czyzewski, and Jones (1996) researched the differences of how mothers and fathers of children with cancer perceive their marriage. The results of this research revealed that poor child health status predicted a more positive attitude toward marriage in fathers but not in mothers. Men rely more on the marriage for social support while women

TABLE 11.4
Family and Personal Relationships

Source of Stress	Reported by
Stress on the Primary Caregiver	Frank, Patricia, Elaine, Matthew, Lynn, Ruth, Joseph
Financial Worries	Frank, Elaine, Timothy, Matthew, Lynn, Ruth
Problems with Siblings	Patricia, Elaine, Lynn
Overprotective Parents	Patricia, Elaine, Timothy, Lynn, Karen
Problems with Personal Relationships	Elaine, Timothy, Matthew, Ruth
Cancer Paranoia	Patricia, Elaine, Lynn, Joseph

tend to have a large social support system outside of the marriage with friends and family. Mothers and fathers both felt positive about their marriage when there were higher levels of commitment and/or lower levels of emotional tension.

In describing their diagnoses and treatments, seven of the nine respondents made particular mention of the stresses experienced by their parents. Most of them recognized that their mothers assumed the major caregiver role and bore most of the burdens of the illness. Elaine remembered that her mother stayed with her constantly, day and night, during her diagnosis and the initial treatments; her father came to visit only on the weekends because he continued to work. When Elaine was home, she slept with her mother in her parents' bed. Matthew also reported that his dad worked but his mother stayed home and took care of him. Lynn and Ruth grew very attached to their mothers because of the amount of time they spent together. Timothy's parents seemed to be the exception; he remembers both parents sharing equally in the burdens of his cancer experience.

It should come as no surprise that many researchers have documented the stresses and strains on marriage that can be brought about by the life-threatening illness of a child: difficulties in adapting, emotional disequilibrium, psychological distress, financial difficulties, health problems, restricted social interaction, alcohol problems, and strained parent–child relationships. The families of the survivors in this book were not immune. Ruth described the uneasiness in her house caused by a persistent bill collector. Money problems dogged Matthew's and Timothy's families, as well. Insurance coverage was a problem for Lynn's family; her father had just changed jobs when Lynn was diagnosed with leukemia. Frank's family was the exception. They were offered, and accepted, community support and fund-raisers to help them make it financially through Frank's illness.

Very few studies have been conducted on the affects on siblings of a brother or sister with ALL or other childhood cancers. Investigations that have been done report that patients' siblings often exhibit jealousy, guilt, chronic anxieties, parallel health fears, anger and resentment, poor school performance, withdrawal, and psychosomatic complaints (Sargent et al., 1995). Many siblings are distressed about family separations and disruptions, lack of attention, focus of the family on the ill child, negative feelings in themselves, and fear of death. Some siblings actually do no better at handling the cancer trauma than the children who actually have the cancer. All of the survivors I talked with mentioned their siblings, but three of the nine described particularly negative feelings their illness created in their siblings. Elaine's brother was 16 years old at the time of her illness; today, he still has problems associated with that time in their lives. Patricia did not discover her sister's jealous feelings until many years after her illness was in remission. And Lynn's younger brother did not understand why Lynn acted the way she did and why she was treated differently from the way he was treated. Lynn's mother found the sibling rivalry very hard to handle.

Like most parents, the parents of the survivors in this book became overprotective. That is the natural order of things—for parents to try to shield their children from pain, or harm, or suffering. This parental protectiveness can be found in many different animal parent–child relationships as well. It is, to some degree, an instinctive behavior on the part of the parent to keep their child safe. However, it is a difficult balance for parents, especially when their child is seriously ill, to keep the child safe and yet let the child experience all of life—the good and the bad. Elaine considered her mom and dad to be "wonderful parents" but agreed that they were very protective of her. Timothy's parents made lots of rules and bribed him if he did well with the medical tests, he would not have to go to school but rather go to his grandma's house to eat. Lynn remembers many restrictions placed on her by her mother. Patricia had the impression that her parents felt they needed to watch over her all the time; restrictions imposed by her parents made her childhood a time with little independence. Karen shared the same perceptions related to how her parents had treated her during her illness and postillness.

The long-term survivor of childhood leukemia has a lot to worry about: making commitments; planning for an uncertain future; problems related to intimacy; worries about sexual relations, sterility and infertility, and pregnancy and possible birth defects; job-related difficulties; and health insurance problems. But high on the list of problems for four of the survivors in this book were difficulties in personal relationships. Elaine recognized what her problem could be: "My problem is I am very giving, sometimes too much. That bothers other people." Matthew also seemed to know why his relationships never worked out: "Every time I have gotten into a relationship or whatever, I have never necessarily wanted to get married. I've come close but it just wasn't right. It didn't feel right. Because it feels like I'm supposed to be doing something else." Timothy married his high school sweetheart and best friend but even after 5 years of marriage, the close relationship he developed with his family when he was ill is a source of stress in the relationship with his wife. Ruth never dated much and feels uneasy about dating. She attributes this feeling to the fact that she was ill during a critical time in her adolescent development. Years later, she still doesn't know how to handle it.

Part of the problem may well be that these survivors are fearful that, because of the cancer treatments they endured, their offspring may be born with deformities and/or disabilities. Matthew believes he is sterile. Ruth knows she is infertile. Patricia is openly worried about having a normal baby. Timothy was terribly distraught during his wife's two pregnancies, worried over possible physical deformities and/or cognitive disabilities.

Conflicts over whether to disclose to people their history of childhood leukemia also continues to haunt many survivors' personal and professional relationships. Matthew's family had always planned to keep his leukemia a secret and, as an adult, Matthew makes it a habit of not disclosing his past illness. He worries about the impact of disclosure on jobs and insurance. Patricia is just the opposite. She makes a point of being honest about her health history when she goes on job interviews.

Cancer paranoia is the common feeling of anxiety, fear, and nervousness that the cancer will return one day. Many pediatric cancer survivors experience this as an aftermath of their illness, and it is a warranted fear. As a result of the toxicity of their treatment, long-term survivors of pediatric cancer face a 20 times greater than expected probability of being diagnosed with a new cancer. Most pediatric cancer survivors can expect continuous medical follow-up throughout their lives. These follow-up appointments involve several painful diagnostic procedures and are approached by patients and their families with anxiety and guarded optimism. Viewed from this perspective, childhood cancer is a chronic medical condition associated with long-term physical, psychological, and social consequences. This kind of "waiting for the other shoe to drop" characterizing uncertainty has been termed the "Damocles Syndrome." Koocher and O'Malley (1981) first introduced the Damocles Syndrome as a psychosocial consequence. They had observed pediatric cancer survivors having difficulties with self-esteem, depression, anxiety, peer relationships, school, and work. The name comes from a Greek legend, a story "told by Cicero about a sycophantic courtier invited by the tyrant Dionysius I to enjoy a luxurious and bountiful feast while sitting beneath a sword suspended by a single horsehair" (Rait et al., 1992, p. 385).

The survivors in this book were not immune to the Damocles Syndrome, even 10–20 years after their childhood cancer experience. Elaine has experienced anxieties of sufficient intensity that she has considered seeing a counselor. Matthew's anxieties reappear each year as he prepares for his annual checkups. Lynn also gets very nervous at checkup time, but her anxiety is not limited to that—she worries every time she feels sick or overtired. Patricia's anxieties about the return of cancer were borne out when she was diagnosed as an adult with cervical cancer. Although the doctors believe she is now fully recovered and in remission, Patricia believes that "it never really leaves you, not ever." Joseph characterizes the feelings as "a great dark shadow." For Joseph, this shadow comes and goes. For Timothy, it is a more constant threat. However, all nine respondents describe in their own words the feeling that the cancer experience is always with them. It is a shadow that they feel will walk side by side with them throughout the rest of their lives. But interestingly, whether they view this "shadow" as a negative or a positive influence in their lives, they merely accept it as a part of their past, present, and future lives. It is a reminder of what they have experienced and who they have become today as a result of it and what it may lead them to be or do in the future.

12

Childhood Leukemia
and School

Without the comfort and love of other human beings, none of
us is very strong. Aligned with others who accept us and support us, we can survive most anything.

—Ann Kaiser Stearns

For school-age children, going to school is a fundamental ingredient of a
normal life. School structures the days and weeks of at least 10 months of
each year. It provides access to peers and teachers. It is where children develop more than just academic skills. School provides learning experiences
for a child's social and emotional development as well. According to
Spinelli (2004), "Returning to school is not only important for maintaining
continuity in their educational program and interaction with peers, but it
is reaffirming and reassuring to patients and their parents suggesting an
expectation that life will go on, that they will have a future" (p. 14).

Childhood cancer interrupts the rhythm of a child's life. For a short
time, it changes life completely. For a longer time, the child, her or his family, and her or his school can feel its effects. It is a time in their young lives
when they must face immense adult circumstances such as feelings of fear
and frequent pain associated with the very treatments that are meant to
save their lives.

The school environment offers children who have cancer an opportunity
to experience life as a student and nat as a cancer patient. It is within the

walls of a classroom that children living with cancer or who have survived cancer can retrieve their childhood. Each child's experience of school is unique. However, within the context of these nine stories we have read remarkably similar reports of the importance of maintaining contact with teachers and classmates during treatment. We have read about their struggle to keep up with schoolwork over the long term, and of the critical role school played in helping the survivors get back to "normal."

According to Keene (1999), sometimes parents do not know what normal is after diagnosis and it may be different from family to family and child to child. She believes normal is what feels right for the family and the child at any given time. Parents need to realize that their child having cancer is not a normal childhood experience. It is not a normal experience within the context of their marriage and the family structure.

Most young survivors report a strong need to return to a normal life, to be treated normally, and to be just like their peers. But they also battle within themselves with concerns of their physical appearance, social concerns of fitting in with the group, and having a deep desire to have those around them understand and appreciate all that they have gone through from diagnosis to survival.

There is very little research to date about how children and their families handle the school environment after diagnosis. Most of the research surrounds issues of finances, marital adjustment, problem-solving and coping strategies, psychosocial issues, emotional distress, sibling difficulties, and family cohesiveness. It is apparent in the research literature that mothers and fathers of children who are diagnosed with cancer undergo many challenges.

There have been very few explorations of parents' views of school and education in the context of a child having been diagnosed with cancer. Spinetta and Deasy-Spinetta (1981) describe the normalizing effect of school on children and their families, but they never mention how the attitudes and perceptions of parents, teachers, and classmates impact the process of survival. A very interesting perspective about school is offered by Martha Askins, Ph.D., clinical psychologist and educational coordinator of the M. D. Anderson Department of Pediatrics: "In addition to school broadening the mind, it also heals the soul for a young cancer patient" (Cancer Wise, 2003).

In this chapter, I draw from the nine stories to illustrate the role of education and school in the survival experience. I begin with the difficulties encountered by the young survivors in maintaining contact with the school and returning to school.

TABLE 12.1
Schooling Variables that Impacted the Survivors

Schooling Variables	Survivors Affected
Schooling during the Initial Stages of Treatment	Patricia, Elaine, Timothy, Lynn, Ruth, Joseph, Karen
Extended School Absences	Frank, Patricia, Elaine, Timothy, Matthew, Lynn, Ruth, Joseph, Karen
Returning to school	Frank, Patricia, Elaine, Timothy, Matthew, Lynn, Ruth, Joseph, Karen
Disclosure to School Personnel	Frank, Patricia, Elaine, Timothy, Matthew, Lynn, Ruth, Joseph, Karen

SCHOOLING DURING AND IMMEDIATELY FOLLOWING THE ILLNESS

School is the nucleus of a child's life.

—Nanci A. Sullivan

For children with cancer, participating in school is an essential part of feeling, and being, cured. School provides children with the necessary ingredients of stability. Going to school is "normal." Social and academic school-related activities provide an important opportunity to normalize, as much as possible, a very difficult and ongoing stressful experience. The child who is denied continued school participation is, in effect, being denied a major opportunity to engage in what is considered normal age-appropriate, goal-oriented behavior. Such interference may lead to a sense of learned helplessness, and may reinforce feelings of hopelessness and despair. Table 12.1 summarizes the schooling variables that affected the survivors.

SCHOOLING DURING THE INITIAL STAGES OF TREATMENT

One of the most remarkable findings to emerge from the stories in this book was the consistent reports from parents about the priority they placed on their child's education even during the most frightening periods of their child's illness. Perhaps, for parents as well as children, focusing on school meant focusing on the future, focusing on survival, focusing on getting back to normal. It certainly appeared as if parents' focus on school helped encourage and balance the relationships, interactions, and feelings within the family unit during this crisis.

Eight out of the nine respondents had parents who really valued the uninterrupted continuance of their child's education, during hospital stays, during convalescence at home, and during subsequent chemotherapy or radiation treatments. Elaine's parents focused on keeping her education a constant priority. When Elaine was up to it, her parents encouraged her to attend the school at the hospital. When she couldn't attend the hospital school, her parents worked with her on schoolwork. Timothy recalls that his parents also kept schoolwork in the foreground; to Timothy the schoolwork was actually a welcome distraction. Karen's parents also worked with her throughout her illness. Patricia's sisters joined her parents in developing a system for helping her to continue her schoolwork, while Joseph's school sent his assignments to the hospital where hospital staff and volunteers would help him in completing it. Lynn and Ruth both depended on their mothers to stay involved with their education.

Extended School Absences

Our nine respondents missed a lot of school from the date of initial diagnosis through to the beginning of the maintenance phase. Depending on the date of the diagnosis, some were out for as little as 6 months and some for as long as one full year. Lynn was diagnosed in December of her kindergarten school year and missed the rest of that school year. After being diagnosed with ALL, Elaine missed most of first grade, from the middle of November through June; in those 7 months, she had several major setbacks such as septic shock, a staph infection, and a collapsed lung. Timothy was also diagnosed with leukemia in November of his first-grade school year and missed the remainder of that school year. Matthew was out of school from January of first grade through to the end of the school year. Ruth missed the latter part of her first-grade year. Frank was in second grade when, in November, he was diagnosed with ALL and taken out of school. His doctors did not permit him to return to school until the last few weeks of the school year.

An intriguing sidebar is that seven of the nine respondents were diagnosed with childhood ALL during the winter months (Lynn in

December, Elaine in November, Timothy in November, Matthew in January, Frank in November, Joseph in December, and Patricia in February). Ruth and Karen were diagnosed in the spring (May and April, respectively). Perhaps, it would be interesting to research the months of the year as to when the majority of childhood ALL diagnoses are made. It could be hypothesized that the majority of diagnoses are made in the winter months due to the many viruses and infections that children usually acquire in school that could greatly affect their immunity systems. When the immunity system is at a point of being in overload and vulnerable, that is quite possibly when cancer cells can erupt.

Returning to School

One of the greatest problems that parents encounter with children who have cancer is reintegrating them into school. List, Ritter-Sterr, and Lansky (1992) reported that children who do not return to school early find it increasingly difficult to reintegrate later. Nevertheless, many parents delay the return to school because they fear it will be too much, physically and emotionally, for their child. And, as the return to school becomes imminent, it is not unusual for both the parents and the child to display some separation anxiety. This anxiety may manifest itself as a series of somatic complaints. The parent responds to these somatic complaints by allowing the child to stay home and not attend school. Then, patterns of absenteeism complicate the reintegration into school even more. Sometimes, the child becomes school phobic and ultimately refuses to attend school at all. However, parents and educators need to be aware that the greatest predictors of psychological adjustment for children who survive cancer are high levels of support from the family, classmates, the school, and the hospitals (Kazak, 1994).

Eight of the nine survivors experienced difficulties in returning to school. Some had minimal problems—though they still remembered the problems years later. Others faced problems that have left a lasting impact on their school memories. While some of the difficulties were related to physical appearance such as no hair and puffiness, psychological issues occurred such as acceptance from classmates. Still others were concerned about their academic careers as a result of being behind the rest of the class or not being able to keep up. However, it was apparent that their school reintegration did pose some serious long-term feelings and thoughts about the experience, thereby reinforcing that school is the nucleus of a child's life.

Disclosure to School Personnel

One of the most difficult decisions parents faced during the cancer ordeal was who to tell about the illness. And disclosure is more than telling the truth to the child. Disclosure also extends to telling family members, friends outside of the family, neighbors, colleagues, school personnel, and the child's classmates and schoolmates. In several of the stories told here, medical personnel offered little advice and had no communication of any sort with the schools of the survivors. The task of communicating about cancer and monitoring the child's medical progress usually fell to the mother. Today, however, there are often hospital liaisons who help the families with communication from hospital to home to school.

For some parents, disclosure was not an issue; they told everyone. Frank's parents maintained open communication with his teacher through his illness, and for years, the principal and teachers in his school inquired about how he was doing. Frank simply assumed that everyone at his elementary school knew about his illness. Elaine's mother and Timothy's mother also communicated freely with their children's teachers and counselors.

But some parents did more of a juggling act by selecting who would be told about their child's illness. Patricia's mom kept the truth from Patricia, but she managed to let everyone know at school. It was the same with Lynn. Her mother did not tell her very much about her condition, but she did disclose all the necessary information about Lynn to her teachers, principal, and school nurse.

The truth about Ruth's health came out when school medical forms had to be submitted. After submitting the forms, Ruth's mother would usually call the teacher at home and explain Ruth's abilities and limitations. Most teachers just took the information in stride. But Ruth remembers one teacher who seemed traumatized by it and seemed to avoid contact with Ruth after learning about her illness. Both Joseph's teacher and the school nurse knew about his illness, but Joseph found it very difficult to admit to anyone at school what he was going through at the time. So both his teachers and the school nurse were told not to inform any of the children in the school about his illness.

Many parents worried about the detrimental effects of telling others about their child's serious condition, taking the risk of having their child thought of as "different." When Karen and her family moved to a new neighborhood after her second-grade year, her mother did not tell the teachers in Karen's new school about her having survived cancer. Karen thinks that made third grade even harder for her.

ONGOING SCHOOL-RELATED PROBLEMS

School helps children maintain a balance within their psychosocial selves. School provides a context for the development of children's feelings of self-worth. School is a child's "social world" where she or he can learn to interact and to deal with negative and positive relationships and situations. School is where friendships can be formed that can last a lifetime. School is where survivors prepare for their futures just as their healthy classmates do.

Attending school remains the foremost task in the lives of young and adolescent children. It anchors their lives and serves as a primary influence for academic and social development. Returning to school following diagnosis and during treatment should be considered a milestone for young survivors. School reintegration readily serves as the primary method by which psychosocial cure is approached and with this cure comes the internal sense of returning to a "normal life"—to a sense of "balance" after such uncertainty and turmoil. For any child, returning to a normal life and regaining balance would include attending school—learning, interacting, growing, and developing.

But the mere act of returning to school does not offer a comprehensive solution to psychosocial cure. Survivors, parents, and teachers are often apprehensive and worried about school reentry because they must deal with uncertain outcomes or consequences of surviving childhood cancer. The success of school reintegration depends on the preparedness of school professionals and the collaborative opportunities afforded them in their efforts to promote normalcy for young survivors of childhood cancer or other serious or chronic illness in the classroom. To keep school a positive experience for cancer survivors takes careful planning; systematic training for teachers, staff, and children; and general preparedness to meet the needs of each individual child at school. For most of the survivors in this book, none of these elements were in place.

Of course, not everything about going back to school was unsettling for the storytellers. Eight of the nine respondents reported very positive school experiences that they associated with their illness. Sometimes it was a special teacher, a tutor, or a classmate who made the difference. Sometimes it was just having someone recognize what extraordinary effort and maturity was required from each of them to continue to participate in school and other activities.

Five of the nine respondents viewed school as providing them with a sense of normalcy during their illness. Some saw school as a "security blanket," a psychological feeling that they would not die if they were in school. Some saw school as a "distracter" that helped them focus on social and learning activities instead of dwelling on their disease and treatment. For all of them, it was a constant act of juggling to retain some form of balance or normalcy in their lives during a serious illness. Table 12.2 describes a set of school problems experienced by survivors during and after treeatment for leukemia.

Continuing Attendance Problems

Once they have returned to school, children with leukemia who are undergoing maintenance therapies tend to have higher than average rates of absenteeism. List et al. (1992), in a study of 39 young adult long-term survivors of childhood cancer, reported that in the year of diagnosis the rate of absenteeism averaged nearly 40 school days. Also, in the year after diagnosis, children were still missing an average of 37 school days, about 1 day a week. Even if a child misses 1 day of school, that child has missed a lot academically and socially. Other researchers have found similar patterns and have reported that even after the survivors were off of all therapies and their medical visits were minimal, their teachers believed that absenteeism continued to be a serious problem.

Some of the reasons for school absences included the obvious: side effects of treatments or time needed for medical procedures such as spinal taps and bone marrow biopsies. But beyond these reasons, there are issues

TABLE 12.2
School Problems Experienced by Survivors

School Variable	Survivor Affected
Continuing Attendance Problems	Frank, Patricia, Elaine, Timothy, Matthew, Lynn, Ruth, Joseph, Karen
Peer Relationships	Frank, Patricia, Elaine, Timothy, Matthew, Lynn, Ruth, Joseph, Karen
Disclosure to Peers	Frank, Patricia, Elaine, Timothy, Lynn, Ruth, Joseph
Teachers as Tutors	Frank, Elaine, Timothy, Matthew, Ruth, Joseph, Karen
Retention versus Promotion	Frank, Patricia, Elaine, Timothy, Ruth, Lynn

such as parents' uncertainty, anxiety, or overprotectiveness, and the children's anxieties, feelings of isolation, poor self-image, or embarrassment over hair loss and weight gain.

The respondents in this book returned to school for the duration of the maintenance phase of treatment with intermittent absences for doctor's appointments and medical procedures. All of the respondents had significant school absences related to the induction and intensified treatment phases of their illness. Elaine's absences during second and third grades were minimal and usually centered on doctor's appointments, a treatment, or a medical procedure. But then she missed all of fourth grade because of a chicken pox outbreak that could have been fatal for her (even though she was considered cured of cancer). Timothy returned to school at the beginning of second grade but he was absent frequently (1 day per week) for treatments or doctor's appointments. His treatment regime, and his high rate of school absences, lasted for 5 years. Patricia could not remember much about school absences, but she did remember being sick from the drugs and suffering from migraine headaches; she assumed that meant many days out of school. Lynn also reported several intermittent absences once she returned to school and over the next 4 years of treatments. But Lynn was not only out for medical visits and a very serious bout of chicken pox; she also did not want to go to school. Ruth went back to school at the beginning of second grade, and was on maintenance treatments during second grade through fourth grade. She felt very stressed because she was always trying to catch up. Then, she missed a semester of her ninth-grade school year due to a bone marrow transplant and peripheral problems associated with the transplant, for example, facial shingles. She found it particularly hard to come back to school after that.

Peer Relationships

Several researchers have reported behavioral adjustment and social competence problems that are related to surviving childhood cancer. Survivors usually participate less in activities, have trouble making and keeping friends, and demonstrate behavior problems. They may be less sociable and have trouble getting along with classmates.

So it was with all but one of the survivors in this book. Frank and Elaine reported feeling like they just did not fit in. Karen and Lynn felt different. Joseph was ashamed of his hair loss and hated the fact that he could not wear a hat in school.

Contributing to the strain on peer relationships was the special connection many of the cancer survivors developed with their teachers. Elaine remembered that students were jealous of the teachers' attention her illness brought her.

Disclosure to Peers

What should you tell the other kids? How much do they need to know? Do they need to know anything at all? The survivors in this book were not of a single mind about these questions. Some wanted their classmates to know about what they were going through—the illness, the treatments, and the side effects. Others did not feel comfortable giving out any information at all. And a few were, themselves, not aware they had leukemia and therefore could not discuss anything with their classmates. Each family dealt with disclosure to classmates in a different way.

Patricia believed that keeping her friends in the dark was the only way to keep them as friends. So, she never discussed her illness, even with her best friend. But "ignorance" often led peers to inappropriate behaviors. Ruth was the only child in her second-grade class not invited to a birthday party because, she thought, the girl's mother had the mistaken idea that Ruth's illness was contagious. Elaine believed that the teasing she had to endure from classmates was a function of their ignorance. Timothy learned to make jokes about his illness and its side effects in order to cope with the peers who made him the center of their jokes. Lynn had no friends to invite to her Make-A Wish Foundation award event because she had not told anyone about the nature of her illness.

Teachers as Tutors

For all of the respondents, teachers played an important role in their lives because school and classmates were often a source of pain or discomfort. During their time out of school after the initial hospitalization, the children's link to school was teachers or tutors. Frank's contact with his teacher at home maintained his relationship with school; that in turn helped Frank reintegrate back to the classroom without any major difficulties. Timothy had a home tutor who helped him stay in contact with his school life while he was at home and even after he returned to school. Timothy's teachers were helpful with more than schoolwork—they provided him with someone to talk after school to and talking to his teachers made things a little bit better for him.

After Elaine returned home from the hospital, she had a home tutor for the last month of school. Then, during the chicken pox epidemic in her school, she was again assigned homebound instruction. Elaine thought she developed a very special relationship with her teachers that persisted throughout her school career. Matthew also felt close to his teachers. He was tutored by one of the nuns at his Catholic school who treated him "like a little angel." Ruth, on the other hand, thought that her teachers sometimes tried too hard, and in the end made things more difficult for her.

Retention versus Promotion

When considering children who have high rates of absenteeism (as is often the case for a child with a serious chronic illness like cancer), the question of grade retention often emerges. Research has shown that 26–47% of childhood cancer survivors are retained in a grade (Mulhern, Wasserman, Friedman, & Fairclough, 1989). Madan-Swain et al. (1998) shared the following statistics from their research that included 47 children and adolescents from 5 to 22 years of age: more than one-third of these students receive part-time special education services, 7% were eventually placed in full-time special education programs, and 8% of the children met the criteria for a learning disability.

Frank, Elaine, and Timothy had very definite views concerning retention. They were very much against it. For these respondents, grade retention was viewed as a punishment for having a disease and for surviving it. They felt it would have been devastating.

In contrast, Patricia and Ruth both wished they had been retained after their early cancer experience. Both believed that had they been retained, their learning problems would have been diminished. Lynn's mother also felt she should have had Lynn retained in kindergarten, to give her just that little bit of extra time to catch up.

COGNITIVE (NEUROLOGICAL) EFFECTS

The most investigated area of research concerning long-term survival of children with ALL is the cognitive effects posttreatment. Many researchers have documented that children who were administered dual systemic treatment (chemotherapy and cranial irradiation) showed a decline in visual-spatial IQ, quantitative abilities, attention or concentration, impulsivity, mathematics, motor speed, timed performance, reading comprehension, spelling, memory, spatial processing, planning ability, and abstract thinking. Sometimes the decline in functioning was evident immediately; sometimes it emerged as late as 10 years posttreatment. Many researchers at the 4–5-year follow-up have found significant declines on intelligence test scores. Children less than 7 years old at diagnosis and treatment tend to exhibit greater declines on tasks measuring quantitative abilities than children older than 7 at diagnosis (Mulhern, 1994). Overall, there is considerable consensus that children who survive leukemia show a decline in cognitive functioning that can be directly related to their cancer treatments. According to Mulhern (2003), there is "A huge variability in academic performace of children with learning disabilities after treatment . . . Modifications to the survivor's environment (tutoring, enriched educational materials at home, and teachers skilled in identifying and helping children compensate for their deficits) can increase the survivor's academic achievements" (p. 5).

All nine survivors in this book reported learning difficulties posttreatment. Whether their difficulties came from the treatments or the absences or a combination of both, it is hard to predict. It needs to be noted that their learning problems might have occurred even if they had not had childhood cancer and its treatments. However, given the extensive and consistent research on posttreatment effects on learning and attention, it is safe to conclude that the difficulties they reported could be attributed to their cancer experience. (See Table 12.3.)

TABLE 12.3
Cognitive Difficulties Experienced by Survivors

Cognitive Area	Survivor Affected
Attention/Concentration	Frank, Patricia, Timothy, Elaine, Lynn
Memory Difficulties	Frank, Patricia, Timothy, Matthew, Lynn, Ruth, Karen
Math Difficulties	Frank, Elaine, Matthew, Lynn, Ruth, Karen
Reading Comprehension Difficulties	Frank, Patricia, Timothy, Lynn, Ruth

Attention/Concentration Difficulties

Eight of the nine respondents commented that their attention/concentration had been affected during and/or after the treatments for ALL. Frank remembered that he could not concentrate when he returned to school after surviving the cancer. Timothy talked about his inattentiveness, about being distracted and always trying to "catch up" in school because of his inability to concentrate related to upcoming medical tests. Joseph stated he had concentration problems during treatments while being in school. Elaine complained of attention and concentration problems at age 15, 10 years after she had completed her treatments.

Many of the survivors found that their attention problems persisted into their adult lives. Patricia reported that her attention wandered when she tried to read the newspaper, and that she frequently lost her place. Ruth rediscovered her concentration problems when she underwent testing at the local Bureau of Vocational Rehabilitation.

Memory Difficulties

Memory problems were reported by seven of the nine survivors. Frank, Patricia, and Lynn all thought their reading comprehension difficulties might be the result of poor short-term memory. Matthew reported having a hard time remembering people's names or remembering what someone had asked him to do. Timothy complained that he had a really hard time memorizing anything. Karen focused on her difficulty in committing the multiplication facts to memory. Ruth talked about her need for multiple repetitions to remember things.

Math Difficulties

Another area that research has acknowledged as an acquired deficit in children surviving ALL and its treatments is in mathematics. Six of the nine respondents identified themselves as having problems with certain mathematical abilities. Karen thought her math difficulties began as early as third grade. Frank and Matthew both admitted candidly that they were not very good in math. Elaine talked about specific difficulties in learning to tell time. Lynn struggled with story problems. Ruth was unable to carry out complex mental calculations and relied heavily on a calculator or pen and paper to decipher a math problem.

Reading Comprehension Difficulties

Five respondents discussed having reading comprehension difficulties. Frank was not sure if his poor reading comprehension was from lack of concentration or a deficit in short-term memory or a combination of both. Timothy had to read and reread a passage several times before he could understand it. Patricia had a pronounced reading disability that has haunted her and limited her employment options well into her adult life. Lynn received remedial reading assistance in elementary school for 5 years, but her reading comprehension problems persisted through middle school, high school, and college. Ruth's reading problems were sufficiently severe to earn her a diagnosis of dyslexia through the Office of Vocational Rehabilitation.

Part III

Looking Ahead to a
Brighter Future

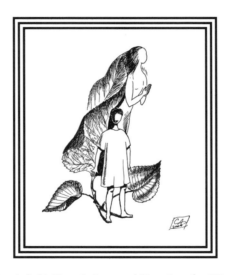

Child to Adult: Surviving and Praying for Normalcy

13

Recommendations for Improved Educational and Psychosocial Outcomes

Preparing a . . . [life-threatened] child for the future by sending
him to school, giving him music lessons, asking him what he
wants from life, is making him like [normal] kids, which is
what he wants most of all, and if research continues, who
knows—he may well have that "fanciful future."

—R. A. Schweers

Children with cancer must deal with terrifying adult circumstances, horrific
pain, and unsettling fears in themselves and in everyone around them. Survival takes courage, and stamina, and good luck. It is a tough road. But the
lesson to be learned from the stories told in this book is that there are ways
that the road can be made a little easier to travel.

The young people I interviewed were most eager to talk when they
learned that they would have an opportunity to make recommendations to
others going through the cancer ordeal. In this chapter are recommendations, focusing specifically on ways of optimizing the school environment
of the pediatric cancer patient. Why focus on school? The answer is school
offers an escape. School can be the stable and normal part of a cancer patient's daily life. School can provide a safe arena of activity and interaction.
Within the walls of a classroom, children battling cancer can retrieve some
of their childhood and, hopefully, be able to form positive social relationships with children of their own age, while at the same time continuing

their education. School gives them a chance to engage in opportunities and activities that seem normal in an otherwise unfamiliar and chaotic world.

With today's medical and technological advances, the classroom teacher who has responsibilities for teaching a child who has a life-threatening illness will not be the exception. More and more children are now surviving leukemia and returning to school in the early stages of their treatment, it is important to help educators, medical personnel, and families make that reintegration to school as successful as possible, to maximize the potential, abilities, and development of the young cancer patient. We must attend to the educational needs of these students because they are a fast growing population in the school community. Following are my recommendations on how to accomplish this task.

From the very beginning and throughout the cancer battle, keep education a part of the child's life. All nine respondents believed that a continued focus on education, even in the hospital, was vitally important to the child as well as to the parents. Educational activities could be very simple, such as reading a story or playing a math flash card game, or more complex, such as working on homework or maintaining computer connections to the classroom. Whatever they are, they help parents and children focus their attentions, however briefly, on something familiar and productive. Educational activities make both the child and the parents hopeful of a future.

Of course, there are many factors that will influence whether a child, in the hospital and undergoing intensive treatments for leukemia, will be capable of attending to schoolwork. All nine of the participants in this book testified that it is quite feasible for children to do schoolwork at the hospital, but some children may simply be too ill in the initial stages of treatment to complete any schoolwork. Usually during the first weeks of treatment, it would be impossible to think of doing schoolwork with the child because the child is too sick and the family, including the child, is under a lot of emotional and psychological duress and anguish. However, significant advances in medicine now make it possible to control the nausea and/or diarrhea that often accompanies chemotherapy, so the more limiting factor may be parents' attitudes about the importance of maintaining an active interest in educational activities. Parents play a pivotal role in determining if and when educational endeavors should be pursued.Our survivors suggest that schooling resume as soon as the child is capable of doing schoolwork, and that the benefits will be not only educational but psychological as well.

Do not try to do everything yourself. Work with the school to get hospital and homebound instruction through regular visits from a teacher or tutor. Another recommendation made by all of the respondents was that a hospital and home tutor through homebound instruction be made available for the child with cancer and any other serious childhood illness. They were quite emphatic about this because of the positive psychosocial effects these individuals had had on them at the time of their illness. Each survivor had been out of school from 6 months to 1 year. Even when they eventually returned to school on a full-time basis, many worried about their continued high rates of absenteeism due to doctor's appointments, medical treatments, or illnesses related to their disease and/or treatments. All nine survivors thought that a tutor was a vital and crucial link to keeping school an active part of a child's life.

Some children with cancer may feel too ill or emotionally upset to deal with schoolwork. On the other hand, according to Ann Bessell (2001), "there is a dearth of research evaluating the effectiveness of homebound or hospital-based instruction, often getting back into the normal routine of academics and getting their minds off their illness and into the normal business of school can be an important mental diversion, provide some routine and normalcy to their lives and help them to envision a future and life after cancer" (qtd. in Spinelli, 2003, p. 60).

A tutor provides a bridge to school for both the child and his or her family. A good tutor plays a very meaningful role in the child's life and in the life of the entire family. The tutor's involvement accomplishes more than just teaching the sick child educational concepts or skills. The tutor brings the three environments—home, school, and hospital—into some semblance of balance and normalcy for all concerned.

Despite how busy and how scared you are, keep lines of communication open among parents, teachers, and the medical personnel. The need for open and clear communications among all the various parties involved with the ill child was clearly articulated by all the respondents. But they also recognized that communication is sometimes complicated by the fact that some parents are reluctant to face or disclose the nature and severity of their child's illness. Outsiders can react fearfully to someone with cancer, as if it were a contagious disease (which it is *not*). People close to the family may, inadvertently, give the impression that they do not want information because of their own personal fears of serious illness, or because they fear being asked to help and being held accountable for their action or inaction. Parents may believe that talking about the illness will expose their child to pity or scorn. The issue of disclosure is also complicated by concerns about confidentiality.

There are two prongs to the issue of disclosure. One is disclosure to the child, family members, neighbors, and friends. The second is disclosure to school personnel. For at least five of the individuals in this book, both prongs of disclosure were problematic. And because families chose not to disclose initially, later disclosure led to major trust issues within the family unit.

The majority of respondents in this book advocated for information to be given to all parties concerned with the child, opening lines of communication among all individuals who are in a position to help the child reintegrate successfully into the classroom. They believed that giving information to people was very important in helping the child cope with the cancer and have a successful school experience. The respondents also felt that the family dynamics were much easier to deal with when everything was "out in the open" and no member of the family had to "walk on eggshells." Everyone in a family is affected by the cancer experience, not just the child who has the disease.

Respondents also felt that the school personnel had a right to know about the medical condition of a particular child in their school or in their classroom. They believed that the teachers should have a complete understanding of the children in their care. Because teachers are held responsible for everything that goes on in their classrooms, survivors believe that complete disclosure regarding treatments, medications, and the side effects was only fair. Disclosure and open communication would be especially important in case of an emergency in which a teacher or school nurse would have to act or make a decision promptly. But disclosure was also considered essential in helping the teacher better serve the child's academic, psychosocial, and emotional needs.

Despite this urging for disclosure, survivors also believed that parents had to feel comfortable disclosing information about their child's cancer and had to be assured that their rights to confidentiality would be honored professionally by the school personnel, if they chose not to disclose. A mutually trusting and secure relationship needs to be developed among all concerned for the benefit of the child.

One way of facilitating disclosure would be for the teacher to initiate contact with the parents concerning the child's disease, treatment, school-related matters, and, when it is time, reintegration. Also, the teacher could request permission from the parents to contact the child's doctor if the parents felt uncomfortable discussing the medical issues related to their child.

It is likely that parents are juggling so many stressful issues related to the child that communication between the parents and the teacher may become secondary. If the teacher makes the initial contact out of sincere concern for the parents and child, perhaps the parents would be more receptive to open interaction with the school. This initial contact from the school could open a new window, which over time might open a door to positive interaction among all the involved parties with the child.

If after the initiation is made by the teacher the parents appear apprehensive and shy away from a discussion, the teacher should employ one of the following two suggestions. The teacher could either stop the interaction altogether in a respectful manner to ensure the family's privacy, or the teacher could, in a calming and reassuring way, stress to the parents the importance of communication at this time between the parents and the school. The teacher could share with the parents that the school should be an added support system for them as well as for their child. It needs to be noted that the teacher should have support from the principal, school psychologist, school social worker, school nurse, and the guidance counselor. Any of these individuals could contact the family as well.

Teachers and classmates will need to be educated. Find resources that can provide that education. It was apparent to all nine survivors that to make the reintegration process successful and less stressful for the child who is ill, teachers and peers need to learn more about the disease and its treatments. They need to have the opportunity to ask questions so they can feel comfortable, as well as prepared, for the child's reentry into the classroom. Elaine shared, "It would be a wonderful thing to have someone come in and talk to the kids at school and explain to them. It would help too if someone spoke with the child."

It is imperative as well that the teacher be instructed about the child's medications because many medications have side effects that might have to be accommodated in the classroom. For example, it is widely known that one common side effect of prednisone is a significant increase in appetite. The teacher may have to make special arrangements to permit the child to have snacks. Other cancer drugs (for example, vincristine) may cause the child to lose his or her hair, to fatigue easily, or to have abdominal pain. The teacher should be alerted that the child may feel self-conscious, or may fall asleep at his or her desk, or may complain of a stomachache. Other drugs (for example, methotrexate) may cause diarrhea, sores in the mouth, joint pain and swelling, coughing, a rash, and so forth. To control side effects, the child may have to eat small, frequent meals (including dry crackers), or drink carbonated beverages, or eat tart foods like lemons or pickles, or be excused from playground or gym class. Some students may also be taking antibiotics, many of which cause stomach cramps and diarrhea; these students may need to have open rest room privileges during those treatment regimes. This would prevent an accident that would result in extreme embarrassment and humiliation in front of a child's peers. Finally, an outbreak of chicken pox can be a life-threatening situation for some children undergoing treatments for cancer; the teacher needs to know to report immediately cases of chicken pox to the parents and/or the school nurse.

Clearly, it is not enough to tell the school only that the child has cancer, or to give extensive generalized information on radiation, chemotherapy, bone marrow transplants, and other aspects of treatment. Instead, the information must be continuous, child specific, and education related. Only when teachers and other school personnel know what to expect, can they come up with positive alternatives for the student in their care.

School personnel cannot be expected to ensure that the chronically ill child will be successful in learning and socializing in school without being informed, guided, and listened to by those surrounding the child (for example, doctors, psychologists, social workers, and parents). Conversely, doctors also must take an active role in learning how the child is doing educationally. Doctors need to know about the school difficulties of reintegration during treatments and posttreatment. Educational personnel also need to learn enough so they can notify the physician whenever the child demonstrates atypical behavior. If doctors are not told of any difficulties the child is experiencing, how are they to know that something may need to be changed? Educational personnel and medical personnel need to work collaboratively to make reintegration into school successful for the child and his or her classmates, parents, and teacher. The issues of a child surviving cancer not only encompass medical difficulties but educational issues as well. It is time that these two disciplines work in synchronization, not as separate entities, for the long-term benefit of the child.

In opening a channel of communication with the child's teacher, it is important to be sensitive to the teacher's own fears and concerns. She or he may have had negative experiences associated with the disease, or may even be struggling to accept or handle a life-threatening illness or death in their own life. Perhaps, the teacher may be a survivor of cancer and therefore finds it hard to deal with in her or his classroom. As Spinetta and Deasy-Spinetta (1981) point out, the very presence of a child with cancer in the classroom stimulates reflection and concern among school staff not only about the child's future but also about their own personal feelings and attitudes. Teachers may need time and opportunity to discuss their own feelings before being able to deal with the feelings of the child and his or her parents and classmates. It might be helpful to make counseling available either through health care professionals dealing with the child, through the school system offering guidance from the school psychologist, or through the educational/medical liaison if one should exist. The teacher should be instructed in coping strategies and problem-solving skills related specifically to having a child who has cancer in her or his classroom. Compassion, understanding, sensitivity, and acceptance are an important commodity for everyone, but most especially for the child's teacher.

Treat the child in an age-appropriate way, including the use of normal disciplinary procedures. Being sick is hard for the child, the family, and the adults and children at school. Often a seriously ill child's overt behavior is a way of compensating for his or her psychological or emotional loss of control. It may well be that behavior is the only thing a child can control in his or her life during the illness. Acting out is the child's way of releasing the feelings of helplessness he or she is facing due to the difficult circumstances. The ability to start and then stop a temper tantrum restores in the child a sense of control. Nevertheless, at home and at school, it is helpful to everyone if limits are placed on inappropriate behavior. McDougal (1997) stated, "The child may show academic and behavioral problems that are a result of treatment, and thus the teacher will need to adjust to the needs of the individual students. However, the teacher should maintain appropriate expectations regarding the child's schoolwork" (p. 8).

Discipline should be meted out fairly, but even sick children should not to be allowed to get away with temper tantrums or other inappropriate behaviors. Sometimes, when a child has a serious illness, everyone "spoils" the child in trying to overcompensate for such a terrible and "unfair" situation. Of course, discipline does not equate with using physical punishment (as was used with Timothy and Matthew); it could mean making use of time-out especially with an ill child. Instead, using time-out (a maximum of 1 minute for each year of the child's age) or withholding things important to the child such as TV time may help shape the child's behavior, as would the use of positive reinforcements (rewards) for acting more appropriately.

It is important to provide the child with "choices" during this difficult time. When a child is given choices, he or she may feel some control in their lives. Timothy said it simply, "It is important when a child is struggling to survive that they have choices in their lives. I chose where I wanted [them] to take the bone marrow from or what finger I wanted them to prick for blood. It gave me confidence. I choose to wear a hat instead of a wig." The following are some examples of choices to give the child at home: What would you like to have for a snack? When will we do schoolwork, before dinner or after dinner? What sounds good to you for dinner? The following are some examples of choices that could be given to the child at school: Do you want to write your spelling words or spell your spelling words to a peer for practice? Do you want a peer helper? Do you want to work in a group or by yourself today?

It is also important to remember that if medication is causing the ill child to act inappropriately (that is, the behavior is not under the child's voluntary control), then disciplining will do neither of you any good. Under those circumstances, it is best to simply remain calm and understanding, and just take care that the child does not harm himself or herself or anyone else. Teachers and parents can only decide how to discipline if they understand the illness and the side effects of the medications, although even then it is difficult to distinguish between the normal manipulations of a youngster and the behaviors that cannot be controlled due to medication. The peers in the classroom will be extremely perceptive in observing how the teacher reacts to and handles any outburst from the child.

Prepare classmates for their friend's return to school. Every child needs to feel a part of the school environment. Extended absences make that hard. The cancer survivor who returns after weeks or months away from class will need help in making the transition back go quickly and smoothly. Teachers, classmates, and the child will have to work hard at this.

It may be a good idea for the class to stay "connected" with the child while the child is in the hospital or at home. The class could write letters, make cards, and/or draw pictures that could be sent to the child. The class could make a cassette tape or a video to send to the child so the child's classmates and the child stay connected, making reintegration easier on both the classmates and the child upon his or her return to school.

Acceptance starts with the teacher. It is important that the teacher attempt to create an accepting and safe atmosphere for the child, one in which the child does not feel as though the disease and its treatments have caused fear and discomfort among teachers and classmates. The teacher will need to balance tendencies to protect and control with the need to let the child become a regular member of the class. The classroom is a microcosm of the outside world, and the teacher is the central and instrumental figure who sets the tone of that environment. The teacher's display of tolerance and acceptance will be contagious and will hopefully spill over to a child's life outside of the classroom.

But modeling tolerance and acceptance will not be enough. Teachers also need to find ways to teach their students about what their classmate has been experiencing and what they can expect when he or she returns to school. Teachers, school nurses, school psychologists, guidance counselors, and school social workers should be knowledgeable enough to discuss or share information with the child's classmates—so someone has to communicate the information they need about leukemia, treatments, educational and psychosocial implications, and physiological side effects. Educational personnel are neither medical doctors/pediatric oncologists nor hospital psychologists, and yet they could easily become the central figure in helping the child and his or her classmates deal with the emotional and psychological consequences of cancer. Teachers know all too well that how they handle a situation in the classroom can have a lasting impact on all those involved in that educational and social environment.

It would certainly be useful if there were someone in the school who had both a medical and an educational background to serve as a resource and support for the teacher, to explain to classmates about their peer who happens to be ill. However, such individuals are rarely part of the staffing of a school.Instead, the teacher should seek out all the available pamphlets and materials from the American Cancer Society, the Leukemia Society of America, the local Leukemia Society, the National Cancer Institute, the Candlelighters Childhood Cancer Foundation (parent support group), and many other cancer organizations (contact information is provided in Appendix 4). These places will be able to offer basic information about cancer or more specifically about leukemia, treatments, medical vocabulary, and what to expect from the treatments. Second, there are annual conferences that can offer teachers and other school personnel information about childhood cancer, the treatments associated with the specific types of cancer, and psychosocial issues related to childhood cancer (for example, the Council for Exceptional Children and the Cancer Survivorship Conference). Next, a teacher could reach out to community volunteers such as a nurse or a hospital psychologist to be a visitor in their classroom to help communicate to the children on their level about childhood cancer.

Another resource that teachers might find beneficial is a lesson plan that was developed by Peckham (1993, pp. 29–30) for use with elementary children whose classmate has been absent from school due to childhood cancer and will be returning to school soon (see Figure 13.1). This lesson plan can be adapted and formatted for use at any grade level, or generalized to other chronic illnesses. Peckham (1993) suggests that the teacher, in addition to using this lesson plan, have "class sessions that are interactive and encourage children's questions . . . allowing the teacher to clarify misunderstandings while presenting new ideas" (p. 28). During such a lesson, the teacher needs to portray an aura of accessibility so both the child with cancer (if the parent agrees that their child should be present) and the other children in the classroom feel comfortable asking questions or simply talking if the need presents itself. Peckham also stresses that educational personnel must talk to the child's parents about confidentiality and disclosure to clarify what can and cannot be shared. Spinelli (2003) also comments, "Presenting a lesson on cancer, its causes, types, treatment, and the side effects of treatment and assigning students [age-level appropriate] to research related topics can help dispel the myths and provide students with current information" (p. 59).

FIGURE 13.1
A Lesson Plan on Childhood Cancer (Grades 6–10)

Introduction

Usually some members of the class will be aware of their classmate's illness and its seriousness. However, some children may not know or may have heard erroneous information. If you ask directly, "Do you know what cancer is?" most children will nod their heads in an effort to please the questioner. They may well have some notion of emotions associated with the use of the word *cancer* and therefore think they know what the word means. If you take their "yes" at face value and move on, you will have missed a chance to teach and clarify. Most successful lessons start by engaging students and connecting new material with that previously known. This topic is no exception. Therefore, the following sample lesson is in dialogue form, which encourages comfortable interaction with students and teacher.

How many of you know someone who has cancer?

Children usually give examples of adults in their lives who have cancer. They may mention the sick student or other children. Acknowledge each child to understand his or her point of reference and connect the child with the lesson. If no one volunteers, say, "Some kids know adults who have had cancer and died, like a grandmother or uncle."

Did you know that childhood cancer is different from adult cancer?

More adults get cancer than children. Adults get different kinds of cancer than kids. (Students may know that adults get lung, colon, and skin cancers. Children are more likely to get cancers such as leukemias; brain tumors; and bone, lymph, and nervous system tumors.) More children recover from cancer than adults. Even in children, cancer is a serious disease, and some do die from it. But *most* children do get better. The medicines and treatments are different for children than adults. Almost all children come back to school while they are being treated for cancer.

Did you know that there are different kinds of childhood cancers?

Give a brief explanation of childhood cancers in terms of the body system. For example, leukemia is a cancer of the blood (bone marrow makes blood), brain tumors are in the head, osteosarcomas affect bones, and Wilms' tumor affects the kidney. There are also muscle, eye, and lymph node cancers. Any place in the body that has cells can have cancer.

Does anyone know what cancer is?

The body is made up of cells that are constantly growing and doing their special jobs. Cancer cells are cells that grow too much and take the place of cells that should be there doing their jobs. You can make an analogy to weeds growing in a garden. You need to get rid of the weeds. Ask about different ways the children know to get rid of weeds, like pulling them out or spraying them with weed killer. Surgery to remove the cancer is like pulling out the weeds; chemotherapy is like using the weed killer.

The kind of cancer your classmate has is called _____.

It helps to be specific and write the name of the disease on the board. You should talk with the child and parents to learn how much and at what level of detail they wish the class to be informed. Use the printed resources available from the American Cancer Society, the National Cancer Institute, and various disease societies to inform yourself to

the point that you are comfortable using the language and information appropriate for the age and grade of your students.

Do you know how kids get cancer?

See what answers you get. Some children will answer "From smoking
or eating certain foods." If you have gross misconceptions about how
people get cancer, correct them immediately (e.g., "You don't get cancer
from swimming in dirty water"). Take the opportunity to explain that
we know certain things that cause adult cancer, such as smoking, sun-
burn, and poor diet, but mostly we do not know. We do not know how
children get cancer. Stress that it is nothing that the person, his or her
parents, or friends have done. You *can not catch* cancer in the same way
you can catch a cold. It is not anyone's *fault* that a person gets cancer.

**Can you get cancer by sitting next to or playing with someone with
cancer?**

Reemphasize that cancer is not contagious! Children do not catch cancer from sharing sodas or being close to a child with cancer.

Do you know how cancer is treated?

There are three different kinds of treatment for cancer. Sometimes
children need one, two, or all three kinds. Explain that the student is
having surgery and/or radiation and/or chemotherapy, which is appropriate. If the student is present, this is a good time to encourage his
or her participation in describing what is done at the hospital.

Surgery. Ask, "Does anyone know someone who has had an operation?" Often students will tell you their own experiences with stitches,
broken bones, or having anesthesia for surgery. Bring them back to
the topic by explaining that some cancers are taken out by surgery.
The surgery can remove some cancers, but often the cancer cells are so
small and good at hiding that the doctors need to use other things to
stop them from growing (so they do not grow back, like weeds).

Radiation. Ask whether anyone has ever had an X-ray. Usually all the
children will raise their hands. Explain that radiation is like an X-ray
but much, much stronger. It does not hurt, but the patient must lie
very still. The radiation beam is aimed at the exact spot where the cancer is. Radiation stops the fast-growing cells. Sometimes it stops other
cells, too, but they usually start growing again. Introduce the idea that

later you will talk about the things that happen after the treatment—side effects.

Chemotherapy. Ask, "Does anyone know what chemotherapy is?" Explain that chemotherapy is a special combination of very strong medicines that stop cancer cells from growing. Some of these medicines are given like a regular "shot" or pill. Some medicines need to go directly into the blood in a vein using intravenous (or IV) needles. Some children who have cancer need to have a lot of "sticks" with needles, and that can hurt a lot, so sometimes the doctors will put a catheter into the chest. This is a long, thin plastic tube that is surgically inserted into a large vein so that medicines can be injected into it without having to "stick" the skin frequently. The end of the tube is capped and taped off to the child's chest. It causes no discomfort and limits daily activities only minimally.

How do you think the doctors know when the cancer has gone away?

They do tests. That means more needles, blood drawn, fluid taken out of the spine, and urine samples. Ask whether the children have had blood drawn at the doctor's office. Can they remember what that feels like? Emphasize that children with cancer have to be very brave because a lot of things they have to do hurt. Help the classmates appreciate how much hard work it is to get better from cancer.

Do you know what side effects are?

These are other things that happen because of the treatment. Sometimes children look different because of their side effects. One of the main side effects is loss of hair. Children may feel sick to their stomach. They may vomit frequently when they are on certain medicines. They may gain or lose weight. Some children develop mouth sores and find it difficult to eat certain foods. Often children are tired while on treatment. Some medicines may cause temporary problems with balance and walking or handwriting.

Older students can understand the reasons why treatment has side effects. For example, the medicines stop fast-growing cells in the body. Some of the fastest growing cells in the body are the hair and those that line the mouth. Hair cells form a shaft. When they stop growing, the hair falls out. Hair loss usually happens a week or two after the medicines are stopped. Sometimes it comes back just the same, other times it may even be a different color or texture.

Ask the class to understand their friends may be self-conscious about not having their hair and will want to wear a cap, scarf, or wig. Explain that the child certainly will not want to be teased about it. To emphasize this point, ask the class how they would feel if tomorrow they had to come to school looking different or if they had to get glasses or braces. Would they want to be teased?

Try to relate their own experiences to that of the ill classmate. Ask whether anyone has ever had a cold sore or canker sore. What would it feel like to have a whole mouthful of sores? Would there be certain foods they would not eat? Maybe they would only want to eat foods that did not hurt, some medicines that children with cancer have to take cause them to be very hungry and gain weight or retain fluid. Children on treatment do not want this to happen, and it is not their fault. They do not want to be teased about being fat. Emphasize to the classmates that their friend is still the same person even if his or her body looks different. Assure them that after the medicines are finished, their friend will look more normal.

Children on treatment often have to take medicines in cycles. That means that they will have several days when they feel nauseous and vomit frequently but then have good days when they feel better. It is important for the class to learn to take this in stride as much as young cancer patients do. Ask the class whether they have had the flu and been sick to their stomachs. Explain that this is the way the medicine makes children on chemotherapy feel. It is not easy to feel this way, but they can continue to go to school. It helps if their classmates are understanding.

Ask the students what they can think would be helpful to their friend. They may suggest helping the student go to the bathroom or nurse's office, keeping track of classwork or assignments while the student is out of the room, or helping with specific lessons in math or reading.

After a discussion about cancer, ask the class to be special friends with their classmate on the playground or on the bus. They can now be emissaries to tell the other children in the school about cancer and its side effects.

Source: Peckham (1993).

A final resource that might be helpful is the Bibliotherapy provided at the end of this book as Appendix 1. It provides information on books, videos, cassette tapes, and Internet Web sites, as well as a listing of no-cost materials that are currently available to use with children. A synopsis of each of the informational entries with age levels and grade levels has been included to help as a guide in choosing the appropriate material for a given situation or environment. Also, in Appendix 5, you will find a listing of organizations and foundations and further reading material associated with childhood cancer from the Bone Marrow Transplant Information Network.

Help the child deal with classmates and reintegrate into the social fabric of the school. It might be helpful to assign the newly reintegrated child to a peer-partner to help him or her become reacquainted with the school routine, to encourage social interaction, and to help with assignments. This buddy system can serve two useful purposes. First, it would provide the child with academic support when returning to school, and someone to ask questions of, someone to help with assignments, and someone to offer support when the teacher is busy. Second, a strong friendship might develop that would also be helpful for the child with cancer who returns to school. Encouraging the young survivor to participate in ordinary tasks, responsibilities, and school activities might also be helpful. Some of the survivors in this book participated in sports, the band, cheerleading, camps, or student clubs, always with his or her physician's approval.

By following such guidelines, parents not only facilitate a return to the normal routine, but they also show the child that they have an optimistic expectation that the child will survive. Unfortunately, it is often hard for parents to remember what "normal" is and to not be overprotective, which can cause other issues for the child and the family. Returning to the carefree precancer days is not possible; that life has changed. Normal is a moving target—different for every person and family. Normal is what keeps the family alive and planning and moving together to face their individual and collective futures. For some, normal is putting the cancer behind you. For others, it is making it a part of everyday life. For example, Joseph and Karen both commented with enthusiasm about Camp-Can-Do, sponsored through the American Cancer Society. They had attended this camp during their battle with childhood cancer and continued to attend every summer up to the age 18. The camp provided them with normal outdoor activities but also a chance to be with other children who had cancer. Normal is what feels right for now. No one can tell anyone else what normal will be.

Stay vigilant about the child's progress in school. Be aware of possible late-emerging learning difficulties. Children surviving leukemia are usually expected to have an annual checkup with their doctor to track the medical condition of the child through adulthood after remission and cure. All of the respondents reported immense stress related to those visits; they were all fearful of the leukemia returning or the possibility of a secondary form of cancer being detected. Nevertheless, they kept their annual checkup appointments.

A similar annual checkup should be instituted in the educational arena. Cognitive and psychosocial side effects can emerge up to 10 years or more posttreatment. Therefore, an annual meeting can serve not only to track the child's educational progress but also to keep parents and school personnel alert to the possibility that learning problems, if they do emerge, might be associated with the cancer experience. The meeting could also serve as the vehicle for informing teachers from grade to grade so that they are able to communicate any difficulties that may surface at any time. Finally, the annual meeting will allow for regular and thoughtful discussions of grade retention, often a concern when dealing with children who have a high rate of absenteeism (which is often the case for a child with a serious chronic illness like cancer). Respondents in this book discussed the pros and cons of grade retention, but stressed that, in some circumstances, it might have been helpful.

If upon returning to school there is a need for a diagnostic assessment or if there are learning difficulties that require placement of the child into a special tutoring or remedial program, it is important to characterize these events with the child and the parents as positive and not as punishment. Children with cancer already feel as though they are being punished for having the disease and its treatments. The child must not be made to feel that the testing or remedial help is an added punishment for having the disease and surviving it. It must be stressed to the child that nothing they did caused them to need some help when returning to school; instead, schools recognize that children who are ill and miss a lot of school deserve to have extra help. The help might take the form of remedial services, special education services, or a homebound tutor.

The child may be given a 504 Service Plan under the Rehabilitation Act of 1973 that protects the child from discrimination and may help accommodate the child's needs in the classroom. The school may provide a 504 Service Plan due to the child's medical condition that "substantially limits him or her in major life activities," such as the learning process (Public Law 93-112, 1973). The 504 Service Plan can offer accommodations such as flexible scheduling, extended time to take tests, study guides may be given to the child, or tests may be adapted in some way. The 504 Service Plan can also dictate how to handle the medical condition in the classroom such as the child is permitted to eat snacks often, have more frequent rest room privileges, have a water or juice bottle in class, and so forth.

Under The Individual with Disabilities Education Act of 1997, a child who has cancer may be eligible for services under the exceptionality of "Other Health Impaired" due to his or her "limited strength, vitality, or alertness due to a chronic or acute health problems" (Public Law 105-17, 1997). If the child qualifies under the classification of Other Health Impaired through an evaluation process conducted in the school district by a school psychologist with supportive medical information from the child's doctors, the child will then receive an Individual Education Plan (IEP). School district representatives and parents as a team will design a special program with annual goals and objectives as part of the IEP process for the child. The IEP will be implemented in a special education placement, or under the accommodation section of the IEP called "Specially Designed Instruction," the accommodations would be implemented in either the special education classroom or in the regular education classroom with additional services needed to support the child in an educational environment. Under this section of the IEP, occupational therapy, physical therapy, speech and language services, assistive technology services (software programs, laptop computers, access to video or audio equipment), social worker/counseling services, special transportation, and nursing services (if the child has significant medical needs) may be offered to the child. "School policies may need to be adjusted to accommodate the physical and/or psychosocial needs of the student (e.g. the attendance policy, the 'no headwear' policy). Grade level curriculum standards, program requirements, and state mandates may need to be modified in the IEP (e.g. substitute their physical therapy or an alternative requirement such as a research paper on a cardiovascular exercise for the standard physical education graduation class requirement)" (Spinelli, 2003, p. 57).

Whatever is being offered, it is essential that children are not made to feel punished for having missed school, for being behind their classmates in skills or subject areas, and for having learning problems associated with the leukemia and its treatment sequelae.

Make therapeutic experiences available to the child as they are needed.

Offer the opportunity to the child to keep a written journal. According to the *Encyclopedia of Body/Mind Disciplines* (in Adams [2000]), journal therapy is an act of writing down thoughts and feelings to sort through problems and come to a deeper understanding of oneself or the issues in one's life. Unlike traditional diary writing, where daily events and happenings are recorded from an exterior point of view, journal writing focuses on the writer's internal experiences, reactions, and perceptions. Through this act of literally reading his or her own mind, the writer is able to perceive experiences more clearly and thus feels a relief in tension. This has been shown to have mental and physical health benefits.

People have written diaries for centuries, but the therapeutic component of journal writing started in the 1960s. In the 1970s, actual workshops were conducted around the country in therapeutic journal writing. By the 1980s, many public schools began formally using journals in English classes as well as in other curricular areas. Then during the 1990s, researchers started to conduct investigations into the psychological, emotional, and physical benefits of using journal writing. Interestingly, when "the intention for classroom journals was educational rather than therapeutic, teachers noticed that a simple assignment to reflect on an academic question or problem often revealed important information about the student's emotional life. Students often reported feeling a relief of pressure and tension when they could write down troubling events or confusing thoughts or feelings" (*Encyclopedia of Body/Mind Disciplines* in Adams [2000, p. 2]).

Dr. James Pennebaker, a researcher in Texas, has scientific evidence that writing in journals for just 20 minutes at a time over 3 or 4 days increases immunity system functioning. His investigations "indicate that the release offered by writing has a direct impact on the body's capacity to withstand stress and fight off infection and disease" (*Encyclopedia of Body/Mind Disciplines* in Adams [2000, p. 2]).

"Dr. Joshua M. Smyth and colleagues . . . replicated the well-known research model originated by Dr. James Pennebaker, in which [112] subjects wrote intensively for four consecutive days, 15–20 minutes each day, about stressful life experiences. All subjects in Dr. Smyth's study suffered from rheumatoid arthritis or asthma. Four months after treatment, 47% of those who wrote about stressful experiences showed clinically relevant improvement" (Adams, 2000).

Lastly, Adams states that journal therapy has been effectively used for grief and loss, coping with life-threatening or chronic illnesses, recovery from addictions, eating disorders and trauma, repairing troubled marriages and family relationships, increasing communication skills, developing healthier self-esteem, getting a better perspective on life, and clarifying life goals.

If the child is of age to express himself or herself with words or drawings, then it should be encouraged as an outlet for coping with fears and emotions or to document their experience to help other children. In the Bibliotherapy section of this book (Appendix 1), you will find a few selections where children have used these methods in creating a concrete product in helping other ill children deal with the experience.

Ledoux (1993) views journal writing as a highly personal experience that allows an individual to write "where there are few rules . . . honesty being the only one . . . it is where you create a 'word portrait' [of yourself or life]. You will feel free to write your feelings and thoughts. Keeping a regular journal [gives] some people a feeling of released energy that they do not feel in other writing forms. Journal writing can be an important developmental experience for a person" (pp. 138–139).

> Arts for children in hospitals is a wonderful program. It helps so much to have medical staff who understand the psychosocial needs of children. The art activities help to alleviate children's stress by taking them out of the normal routine of the hospital, and promoting expression, interaction, and normal development.
>
> —Marianne Rinaldo, *child life specialist,*
> *Children's Medical Center, Dayton, Ohio*

Offer the child the opportunity to participate in drawing or in keeping an art journal. Art therapy did not become known as a professional career until the 1930s. Psychiatrists became more interested in art as a form of therapy when their patients' artwork began to show a link between the patients' art and his or her emotions and illness. Also, children who usually exhibit a free and spontaneous type of art form were sharing emotional and symbolic communications in this manner. Art therapy can be used as a primary, parallel, or adjunctive therapy. A state legislative update shows that all 50 states of the United States are in the process of professionally licensing art therapists through various bills at the state level. In November 1998, after 15 years, Pennsylvania passed a title bill that includes art, music, and dance as counseling modalities. Ohio art therapists are seeking an amendment to the Social Work and Counselors Bill that would license art therapists by the established board.

In some pediatric hospitals across America, art therapy is growing in popularity. It is another overt form of communication for children and teenagers to express themselves in a nonthreatening way. Currently, at some universities and colleges across the United States, it is now considered a major in the Arts/Education/Psychology Departments. An individual can now become a child artistic therapist. Many hospitals use an art therapist as a way to help the child or teenager handle and express many of the problems associated with having a life-threatening illness. *Art therapy* simply means a child or teenager uses a form of art to express themselves or their lives. There should be a follow-up session by the professionally trained therapist to discuss the piece of art created by the child. Art therapy may include drawing, painting, and constructing a scrapbook, sculpting, or other types of art expression. Sometimes children have a difficult time using words to express themselves, and art therapy is just another creative expressive form in working through difficult feelings and thoughts about pain, fear, anger, or the possibility of death.

Offer the child the opportunity to participate in music therapy. Music therapy is an established health care profession that uses music to address physical, psychological, cognitive, and social functioning. To be a music therapist, one must have a Bachelor of music therapy degree (4-year program with a 6-month internship). After the internship is completed, a therapist must successfully pass a National Board Certification Exam to become a Music Therapist-Board Certified (MT-BC).

Music therapy for children can be seen at schools who educate students with disabilities such as pervasive developmental disorder, one characteristic of autism, which deals with the lack of sensory connections in a child's surrounding environment. Using music with these children tends to stimulate their sensory connections through the auditory modality, and when teachers try to get the children engaged in singing, it helps with their receptive and expressive language development. Music at a preschool level also supports memory in learning, for instance, the alphabet or numbers.

Music crosses all human barriers. It has the ability to make us happy, sad, sentimental, reflective, and peaceful. It can be classical, pop, country, opera, jazz, new age, and so forth. Whatever our interests are, it affects our mood.

When dealing with young children, who are facing the trauma of cancer, music can provide them with an affective connection to their experience. You can often walk the hallways at Children's Hospital and see young children to teenagers playing their CD players with headsets. Perhaps it provides them with a sense of escape from the hospital environment or pain or simply makes them feel better listening to their favorite music while keeping them connected to the outside world.

Music therapy takes playing a cassette tape or CD of music one step further. It puts a human "face" on music, and there is "live" human interaction between the patient and the music therapist. Music therapy can provide to a child who is facing a horrible life experience interaction, not isolation, and free expression. Music therapy can even provide emotional relief to members of the patient's family when the therapist involves family members. Some hospitals have invested in a music therapist, and it might be worthwhile if you are undergoing a traumatic experience such as childhood cancer to inquire about it at the hospital where your child is being treated.

Contact the Make-A-Wish Foundation. The Make-A-Wish Foundation is one of the most charitable and compassionate foundations that make the wishes of children with life-threatening illnesses between the ages of 2 through the age of 18 come true. The organization was founded in 1980. Anyone in the child's life—doctor, nurse, psychologist, social worker, teacher, principal, friend, minister/priest/rabbi, neighbor, family member—can make a request or recommendation to the foundation in their particular city. The Make-A-Wish Foundation follows up the request with an interview with the child and the child's family. Also, a physician must document the child's type of serious illness. The Make-A-Wish Foundation has never failed to fulfill a child's wish. The top wishes usually asked of the foundation are a trip to Disney World (50%), computers, celebrity meetings, Space Camp, and home entertainment centers. The foundation encourages all family members to participate in the child's wish experience. Make-A-Wish is an international nonprofit organization. There are many volunteers who help make the foundation a success.

Lynn, Ruth, and Joseph were all recipients of the Make-A-Wish Foundation during their battle with childhood leukemia. Lynn was granted her wish when she was in the sixth grade. Ruth was given her wish in the fifth grade, and it was a trip to Disney World, Florida, for her and her family. She said the Sunshine Foundation had actually made her wish come true, but this foundation later merged with the Make-A-Wish Foundation. Lastly, the Make-A-Wish Foundation gave Joseph his wish of a new arcade, a radio, and some tapes.

The Make-A-Wish Foundation can provide a child with a serious illness and their family with some wonderful memories during a very difficult time. This foundation can be a great source of support for everyone.

It is very important to add that the western Pennsylvania chapter has established the "Kids' Club" as a support group for siblings of Make-A-Wish children.

Provide the opportunity for the child to attend a special camp for children with serious illnesses. There are various camps for children with life-threatening illnesses in the United States and in some areas of Europe. The two most known camps are the American Cancer Society's Camp-Can-Do and the Hole in the Wall Gang camps started by Paul Newman, Joanne Woodward, and their friend, author A. E. Hotchner in 1988 in Ashford, Connecticut. "Every summer, 800 boys and girls gather at this camp and just have fun in activities such as swimming, fishing, flying kites, riding horses, [as well as] encourage and comfort each other" (Memmott, 1995, p. 27). Hole in the Wall camps serve children with cancer and other life-threatening diseases all over the United States and Europe. Due to the success of these camps, Newman and Hotchner have added new camps: "The Double H Hole in the Woods Ranch in Lake Luzerne, New York, and the Boggy Creek Gang Camp in Lake County, Florida. In April 1994, a castle in Kildare, Ireland was acquired and began a new life as the Barretstown Gang Camp" (Memmott, 1995, p. 27). Newman's Own, Inc., a gourmet food company, supports the funding of the camps.

Two of the respondents, Joseph and Karen, attended and highlighted the experience of Camp-Can-Do. Sometimes there are local camps in a community that are available. Your local cancer organizations may be able to direct you to the appropriate services for your child to attend a special camp at no cost to the family.

Search Internet Web sites for information. Today, the new informational age is exploding with possibilities because of Internet Web sites. These sites are unbelievable sources of information that can be used right from your own home. It can provide you with vast resources to help and support decisions, as well as educate anyone about all areas related to childhood cancer. Please refer to the Bibliotherapy and the other appendices for a listing of some of the available Web sites that may provide a point of origin.

There are also Internet Web sites for children who have cancer. They can access Internet sites on their own computer. One such Web site is "BandAids and Blackboards," which offers practical suggestions for helping children, their parents, and their educators cope with many issues, especially school reentry. However, there are many other Web sites for children listed in the Bibliotherapy section of this book.

Seek out the necessary help and support to confront and handle childhood death and grief in the classroom.

> The death of a child is always, I think, the most somber
> event anyone ever encounters. But it is a tragedy that can
> be compounded, by a second tragedy, the denial
> [that a] death [occurred].
>
> —Frances Sharkey, MD, *A Parting Gift*

Find out all the information you can about the child's illness, treatment program (for example, possible side effects), and status at the time the child is placed in the school/classroom. Talk to the parents and request permission from them to contact the child's primary physician. Do not feel intimidated; simply state that you are calling to collaborate on ensuring that the child receives the best care possible medically and educationally in your classroom. Hospitals and schools must work together so children are able to attend school while having a serious illness. You may be the professional who initiates this relationship first, but it is essential that it be done for the welfare and betterment of the child who is ill. Since children are now surviving cancer, pediatric personnel and educational personnel must bridge this communication gap. Remember with knowledge and understanding come a sense of confidence, acceptance, and calmness.

If you find yourself as a teacher having fears and distancing yourself from the child because of the threat of the child dying, please seek out professional help not only for yourself but for your interactive relationship with the child. Perhaps you are fortunate enough to have a liaison working in your district; if not, seek out the school psychologist or a hospital psychologist, social worker, minister, rabbi, or priest. Even organizations such as the Make-A-Wish Foundation, the Candlelighters Childhood Cancer Foundation, Camp-Can-Do, and Hole in the Wall camps can offer guidance and support. Discuss the issue of disclosure with the family. Remember you are an educator, but that does not mean that you know everything. There is no embarrassment in seeking out individuals, knowledge, or help. A true educator is capable of knowing where to look for resources in educating themselves. There is no shame in reaching out; only shame if you do not because the child who is ill in your classroom and you suffer because of your fear of asking for help. Do not be afraid to talk about your feelings and thoughts with someone—a person cannot judge another person for their honesty.

If a child dies and the child was a part of your classroom, it would be advantageous for all concerned to invite a professional to your classroom to help the children and yourself cope with the experience of death and grief. Of course, you need to discuss this with your school's administration and the parents before inviting someone into your classroom to help you and your students deal with the emotional or psychological issues related with grief and death. (In Chapter 14, I have included a special section entitled, "Grief and Death in the Classroom." This section has been added because this book is all about surviving childhood cancer but there are times when a child may not survive. Even though today the survival rate is 80 percent for childhood acute lymphoblastic leukemia, it still means approximately 20 percent of children do not survive. Chapter 14 will help educators in dealing with the loss of a child in the school/classroom.)

You can call the hospitals in your community or organizations such as the Make-A-Wish Foundation and the National and Local Candlelighters Childhood Cancer Foundation that work with seriously ill children. Hospice may be able to provide you with someone who could help everyone who was involved with the child. Do not feel because you are an adult and a professional educator that you can handle everything in your classroom concerning a seriously ill child.

Recognize that having a child in the classroom with cancer or a chronically/seriously ill child can add to our lives as educators and to our classrooms to learn about caring, acceptance, tolerance, and sensitivity. It can provide children and teachers with some of the greatest life lessons to ever be taught that cannot come out of a textbook. It can also be one of the most rewarding experiences as an educator as far as personal growth in working with children. Children in your classroom will one day face many of these universal issues in their lives as adults, either with family members, friends, or co-workers. What a tremendous preparatory learning experience it could be for children in your classroom if handled properly.

14

When a Child Dies

Some have a lifetime, some just a day
Love isn't something you measure that way . . .

—Alan and Marilyn Bergman

Death is often seen as the end. Yet, to the education field
it offers the opportunity for new beginnings.

—Schnieders and Ludy

In today's schools, we are seeing a shift in the types of children that the public schools and teachers now must receive and educate. One of the most pronounced shifts that can occur in both special and regular education is the group of students called "health impaired" or "medically fragile." Health-impaired can encompass many different medical problems such as childhood cancer, sickle-cell anemia, epilepsy, juvenile diabetes, hepatitis, AIDS, and so forth. Some medically fragile types of disabilities are spina bifida, cerebral palsy, muscular dystrophy, and so forth.

This book has been centered on the premise of cure and long-term survival and the implications surrounding such an outcome. However, it is just as critical that I address the psychological and emotional aspects of the classroom dealing with the teacher, the peers, and the children themselves as related to the possible death of the child and the grief associated with that death.

It is important to highlight here information derived from doctors, researchers, parents, and children themselves that a child actually knows within himself or herself if and when they are dying. Therefore, on behalf of those closest to the child, it needs to be stressed that communication be an important aspect in the child's final days. Oftentimes, a child will attempt to protect those closest to him or her such as parents, siblings, friends, doctors, and so forth, and not discuss what they are feeling inside. Indirect cues are given to caregivers by the child, indicating they do know what is happening to them. Children do this for their caregivers to take the lead and show their comfort with allowing the child to express his or her feelings, thoughts, and fears. Examples of those cues might be a drawing that illustrates the family without the child, statements about giving away favorite toys to siblings or friends, and reflections about memorable times they shared with their family members or caregivers. Some cues are more overt, such as when a child cries or becomes quiet but no one asks him or her why; the child requests termination of treatment but this is ignored by doctors, nurses, or family members; or the child has outbursts of anger and resentment. In any event, regardless of the child's chosen approach to their impending death, the child is going through a natural emotional detachment and withdrawal from the life he or she has known. Often this type of communication allows closure for both the child and the caregivers of the child.

The medical community and the family are not the only caregivers involved with the child. Today, more and more teachers are having to assume that role in working with the health impaired and medically fragile in their classrooms. Being a teacher, working with young children, you never think you will have to deal with a child who is seriously ill and dying. My research and the research of many others have indicated that teachers are not prepared to handle these types of life-and-death crises in their classrooms. Due to their lack of information and preparation, or that they have faced cancer with a loved one or themselves, teachers will often stay aloof from the child emotionally and psychologically.

Even though adult caregivers are supposed to be emotionally and psychologically supportive of a child, often they know nothing about death. This also hinders the communication process. It may be important to be truthful with the child and to state to them that you don't know what death is going to be like, but that you do know that they will not be alone and they will not feel pain anymore.

Classmates who knew the child who died may find it difficult to accept, understand and grieve. In reviewing the literature it is recommended that death be explained to children in a simple and honest manner. Teaching that death is a natural part of the process of living enables the child to view death as a natural part of life (Doka, 1995). The goal is to support children through the grief, not around it, and not to deny it (Doka, 1995). The following are only some of the strategies to use in supporting a child in grief (Staley, 2000): Tell the child immediately about the death; stay close to the child (hug and touch); continue family routines; let the child see you grieve; express your feelings and validate theirs; encourage questions; let them tell stories; talk about memories that include the person who has died; shed tears, and seek counseling if necessary. What follows is the section on grief and death I mentioned at the end of Chapter 13. It was written in 1996 by Christine Schneiders and Robbie Ludy, and I thank them for allowing me to include it in this book. I believe that these authors promote a comprehensive description of the grief processes of children in a school setting if a classmate should die.

Grief and Death in the Classroom*

Abstract

The composition of today's classroom is changing as more students who are medically fragile and health impaired are entering the educational system. With this change comes the increased likelihood that teachers will be confronted directly with the death of a student. These teachers are expected to mourn the death of the student appropriately, assist other students in responding to the death and modify the grieving process for students with developmental levels of understanding death, factors which affect grieving and symptoms of grief demonstrated by children and adults. Recommendations for specific strategies are provided to support teachers during a time of bereavement.

*Reprinted with the permission of C. A. Schneiders & R. J. Ludy (1996). Grief and death in the classroom. *Physical Disabilities: Education and Related Services*, 14(2), 61–74. The references from this article have been incorporated into the References section of this book.

Today's schools serve a more diverse population than any other time in the history of education. Medical technology allows increasingly more fragile children to survive and live longer (Pendergast, 1995). The federal mandate to serve younger children increases the likelihood that these in-dividuals identified as medically fragile will be served educationally dur-ing their life-span. A dramatic rise in cases of infectious diseases results in children with AIDS (Kelker, Hecimovic, & LeRoy, 1994), Hepatitis B and other health concerns (Kaplan, Smith, & Grobstein, 1994) attending public school programs. Additionally, children who experience trauma, such as traumatic brain injury, are included in the educational system. While the life-span of these children is often much shorter than the norm, more and more of these students are becoming part of the general, as well as special, education system.

Although special educators intellectually acknowledge that students may die, the education field generally avoids this reality (Thornton & Krajewski, 1993). Teacher preparation programs seldom deal with topics concerning death and grieving in the classroom (Rosenthal, 1980). Educators have not been prepared for their own emotional response to a child's dying. Support services are seldom available to educators, leaving them to cope alone (Tait & Ward, 1987). At the same time, teachers are called upon to assist other students and family members with their own research to death.

A complicating variable is society's view that persons with disabilities have a less than equal value to that of their normally developing peers. The acknowledgement of the death of an exceptional child is often voiced by others as a blessing and reduction of burden. Survivors are often left with the impression that they should feel a sense of relief rather than loss. This paradox increases the difficulties of survivors who are attempting to cope with the death of a person with exceptionalities (Chomicki, Sobsey, Sauvageot, & Wilgosh, 1995).

Likewise, helping students deal with death is a complicated issue. Just as adult survivors are expected to return to and/or function in the work place, students who are survivors are expected to return to and/or func-tion in the classroom. Teachers are often charged with the task of noting behavioral changes in students that indicate difficulty in adjusting to the loss of a deceased person (Holland, 1993). This task is complicated by in-consistent responses to death from surviving students. The types of re-sponses shown by students are affected by a variety of factors including the student's level of mental and emotional maturity, personal coping style, cognitive awareness of death, experiential background and per-ceived relationship with the deceased. These responses may differ with each student and situation.

Although teachers have curricular opportunities to explore the entire life cycle, it is often not until a death is experienced within the school community that the topic is confronted. This article presents information to assist educators in developing the skills necessary to handle the experience of death as it relates to the child with disabilities. The article focuses on the following factors: developmental levels of understanding, other factors which effect grieving, symptoms of grief for children and adults, and recommendations for helping.

DEVELOPMENT LEVELS OF UNDERSTANDING

As with other developmental milestones, one's ability to understand death appears to continually evolve. For the purpose of this discussion levels of understanding have been categorized into chronological groupings. There is no evidence that students with disabilities understand death in the same manner as their normally developing peers. Educators must remember these levels were identified for children without disabilities and use caution when applying them to students with exceptionalities (Harper & Wadsworth, 1993).

Crenshaw (1990) identified characteristics demonstrated by infants and toddlers (ages 0–3 years) who come in contact with the death of a significant caregiver. Children at this age have a minimal concept of death and few language skills to seek clarification. They require object permanence to understand death and a concept of self to realize separation. These young children often react with curiosity rather than concern.

Eddy and Alles (1983) report that preschoolers (ages 3–5 years) believe that death is similar to sleep and may express concern that the deceased is cold. Death is perceived as a state that is not permanent. At this age children "play dead" frequently.

Between the ages of five and nine, children recognize death as final and tend to personify death as a character (i.e. angel or skeleton). Children at this stage often express the belief one can outwit death. Their interest in the subject is often described as morbid. Although death is seen as final and concrete, children often believe that death does not happen to everyone (Eddy & Alles, 1983). The deceased person is viewed as being able to see, hear and receive messages from the living (Knowles & Reeves, 1981).

As preadolescents (ages 9–13), youths see death as part of the life cycle, conceptualizing the idea that death can occur at any time (Beckmann, 1990). During adolescence this understanding grows; however, the adolescent often challenges death by taking unnecessary risks (Fredlund,

1977). This relates to evasion, another development characteristic surfacing at this stage. Risks may include racing cars, experimenting with drugs and exploring unsafe areas. Adolescents generally hesitate sharing feelings, preferring to mask their grief in this way (Kandt, 1994).

As noted earlier, these levels are based on normal development of cognitive functioning. If an individual has mental retardation, these stages may be delayed or never fully experienced. Wadsworth and Harper (1991) indicated that persons with mental retardation may experience more than one stage simultaneously. They suggest that a lack of understanding of death appears to be related to cognitive development. This supports an earlier finding of McEvoy (1989) who examined 38 adults (26 male, 12 female) with moderate mental retardation about their understanding of death and found that half of this sample did not know if they would die.

Thus, an ever changing understanding of death can be seen as children mature. Professionals and service providers need to be cognizant that children's awareness of death has impact on their development. Because their impact is seen across the lifespan, adults, particularly those in educational settings, must be aware of the various factors which influence a child's understanding of death and demonstration of grief (Webb, 1993).

OTHER FACTORS WHICH AFFECT GRIEVING

Although the developmental stages are of primary importance, other factors must be considered in understanding how a child may react during the grieving process. These factors include, but are not limited to a child's culture, functional ability, relationship to the deceased, crisis management skills, as well as the cause of death, life changing events due to the death and openness of the family system (Feifel, 1977).

During the time of bereavement, the educator must recognize the cultural diversity of the population served and how those cultures have evolved (Goodman, Rubinson, Alexander, & Luborsky, 1991; Munroe & Munroe, 1975; Pickett, 1993). For example, in the Euro-American culture, medical practice has removed family members as active participants in the medical care of the sick. In the past times children often could observe and participate in the birth of a sibling, care of the ill and preparation of the dead as these activities often occurred at home. Industrialized societies have developed specialized professions which have limited or excluded the family's (and particularly the younger members) participation in such activities. Each culture has its own unique mores with members having distinct roles within each life cycle event (Counts & Counts, 1991).

Another consideration for how one expresses grief is the cause of death. People who have the opportunity to prepare for the death event before its actual occurrence can begin to work towards acceptance—generally defined as the final stage of the grieving process. People who are confronted with death without warning often experience difficulty moving through the grieving process (Munsch, 1993). Death caused by natural occurrences such as illness is often more palatable to culture than those from accident or trauma. Likewise, death of the elderly is often more easily accepted than the death of a child.

Although the death of a child is often less accepted, if the child has a disability, a culture may be more likely to view the death as "as a blessing" (Pickett, 1993). Those left to grieve are often expected to grieve differently in quantity and manner. They may also find fewer outlets to express their grief.

When those who are left to grieve have a disability, the process is further complicated. For example, individuals with limited language and social skills may be unable to express their feelings adequately (McDaniel, 1989). Those who are providing support need to be aware that some individuals with disabilities may not know how to conceptualize their feeling within the limitations of their expressive language (McLoughlin & Bhate, 1987; Kloeppel & Hollins, 1989). Others may be able to conceptualize their feelings but, because of physical limitations, may be unable to communicate them. Individuals with disabilities often have limited social circles providing fewer people to help them through the grieving process. Thus, they are limited in the number of and opportunities for expressions of grief (Wadsworth & Harper, 1991). For these reasons, the teacher of individuals with disabilities becomes an essential component to the accomplishment of a successful grieving process.

As previously indicated, the size and structure of one's social network can affect how an individual is able to express grief. Another consideration is the closeness of the deceased to the mourner (O'Brien, Goodenow & Espin, 1991). Traditional roles and titles do not automatically define the amount and expression of grief. For example, one cannot assume that a child will grieve more for a deceased sibling than for a grandparent. Likewise, in the classroom, a student may express grief for the loss of a classmate in a manner that the teacher would not expect.

The literature indicates that there is a relationship between the number of experiences one has had with death and ease with which it is understood.

Persons who have experience with other life stressors besides death will enter the grieving process with a different set of coping skills than the person who is experiencing death for the first time (Beckmann, 1990). Teachers who have had an opportunity to observe a student's reaction to stressful situations may have some insights into how that student will respond when confronted with death.

The response of a student with disabilities to death may be complicated by life changes that accompany the loss. For example, when a parent dies there may be significant change in housing, income and the amount of emotional support the remaining parent is able to provide. Children with disabilities may be removed from the home and placed in a residential facility as a result of a change in the family's ability to maintain the previous support structure. Likewise, an expression of grief may result in significant life changes. Wadsworth and Harper (1991) and Yapa and Clarke (1989) found that individuals with retardation were more likely to display behavioral outbursts related to grief. Both studies reported implementation changes of placement as a consequence of displayed behavior outbursts. Such actions restrict individuals' social network and ability to express grief.

The ability to express grief is correlated to the openness of the family communication system (Beckmann, 1990). Families may expect members to bear grief silently or to express feeling only within the immediate family. The teacher needs to understand different family communication systems and be aware that students may express grief differently (Holland, 1993). A child may need support even though grief is not openly demonstrated while in the classroom setting. Time is another factor influencing the grieving process. Individuals require opportunities to grieve that are characterized in three stages (Backer, Sedney, & Gross, 1992). In the early stage, the child must understand that someone has died and that the child is safe. The middle stage of grieving is defined as a time to accept the loss and explore the relationship. As a part of the final stage, the child's sense of identity is reorganized and new opportunities for relationships are found.

SYMPTOMS OF GRIEF

Teachers need to be aware of the more common symptoms associated with grieving so that they may effectively help students through the grieving process. Just as teachers acknowledge the social value of grieving, they must acknowledge that not all children will demonstrate grieving behaviors, especially in the school setting (Crenshaw, 1990). Children's symptoms of grief may be grouped into three major categories: physical, emotional and behavioral (See Box 1).

Physical symptoms affect bodily function. Most, if prolonged, can affect the health and well being of a child. Although many may not be readily observed, the teacher should be cognizant of those symptoms which may warrant additional concern. Symptoms such as lack of appetite, exhaustion and inability to sleep will have a direct effect on school performance (Helms & Blazer, 1986).

Educators also need to be aware that physical symptoms may differ across settings. Symptoms demonstrated at home may not be demonstrated at school. Likewise physical symptoms demonstrated on the playground may differ from those showing in the classroom. Educators need to maintain open communication with the child's family and other professionals to get a more complete picture of those symptoms demonstrated by the child.

BOX 1
Symptoms of Grief—Children

Physical Symptoms

- Somatic distress
- Difficulty swallowing
- Difficulty breathing
- Need to sigh
- Lack of appetite
- Exhausted feelings
- Difficulty sleeping
- Lack of muscle power
- Empty feeling in stomach
- Hyperactivity
- Tears

Behavioral Symptoms

- Regression
- Assumes mannerisms of deceased
- Changes in roles
- School problems
- Delinquency
- Substance abuse
- Gives away possessions

Emotional Symptoms

- Hostile reactions toward deceased or others
- Replacement
- Idealization of deceased
- Panic
- Guilt (real or imaginary)
- Isolation or withdrawal
- Shock/numbness
- Anger
- Relief
- Loneliness
- Low self-esteem

Emotional symptoms refer to the internal responses of the child. These responses vary from open hostility to withdrawal to a total lack of demonstrated emotion (Eddy & Alles, 1983). Of particular note is guilt which may be real or imaginary. Beckmann (1990) defines real guilt as the attribution of an action (or lack thereof) as the cause for death. Imaginary guilt may occur when the individual believes that his/her personal thoughts were responsible for death.

Unlike emotional symptoms which are internal, behavioral symptoms include responses to death which are observable actions and reactions. These behaviors may be considered as inappropriate, especially when compared to the child's actions prior to the death. Although these actions may be a natural expression of present feelings, the adult may deem the child's behavior as unacceptable. Some behaviors such as delinquency and substance abuse may be attributed to adolescent rebellion rather than grief expression. These actions may be used to displace the expression of grief. In some cases, the student my seek support from delinquent peers to replace the relationship with the deceased (Eddy & Alles, 1983).

Just as it is important to recognize children's responses to grief it is equally essential that teachers know the symptoms of grief for adults. This will help them assist colleagues and family members of students with whom they have contact. More importantly, teachers need to recognize these symptoms which may occur in themselves. These may be clustered into three groups: physical, emotional, and professional (See Box 2).

Physical symptoms for adults may be similar to those experienced by children. These symptoms include somatically related complaints as well as actual physical illness due to a weekend state. Like their young counterparts adults may demonstrate differing symptoms in differing physical settings.

Emotional symptoms relate to the general category of depression causing a lack of motivation and personal involvement to be demonstrated by the adult. In addition, the grieving adult may demonstrate uncharacteristic outbursts such as expressions of anger of tears. Specifically related to the grieving process, the adult may perform a type of mummification whereby artifacts of the deceased are maintained as if the deceased were still alive (Feifel, 1977).

Adults may experience symptoms specifically related to performance of professional duties. They may feel ineffective in their jobs and a lost sense of personal as well as professional control. This feeling may be compounded by a change in job responsibilities due to the death. For teachers, this may result in a demonstration of symptoms often associated with

BOX 2
Symptoms of Grief—Adults

Emotional Symptoms

- Mood changes
- Depression
- Irritability
- Sudden outbursts of anger over minor occurrences
- Small problems are seen as insurmountable
- Relationships with others become difficult
- Crying for no reason
- General feeling of emptiness
- Poor self-image
- Disorganization
- Overly active
- Mummification

Physical Symptoms

- Sleep problems
- Physical illness
- Tearfulness

Professional Symptoms

- Professional feelings ineffectiveness
- Senses of loss of self-control
- Helplessness
- Unwillingness to make emotional commitments

teacher burnout including a decline of emotional commitment to students and the education field (Tait & Ward, 1987).

INTERVENTIONS

Before intervening in the grieving process, teachers must examine their feelings about death (Thornton & Krajweski, 1993). If this self-assessment reveals that the teacher is unable to confront death as a natural part of living or if cultural considerations prohibit the teacher from engaging in open discussion, then alternative methods must be found. The teacher must be willing to acknowledge the inability to handle the responsibility of this topic, and ask a counselor or a psychologist to work with the students.

Teachers should provide an environment where children can feel safe in the truthful expression of their feelings and questions (Berg, 1978; McLaughlin, 1994). To create a safe environment, teachers must utilize accurate and clear language regarding death to avoid misinterpretations by children. Likewise teachers must clarify euphemisms and metaphors related to death when talking with children (Helms & Blazer, 1986). The use of expressive strategies (i.e., storytelling and monologues) may assist educators in helping students become aware of how to appropriately respond to grief. Teachers should present information systematically, progressing from basic to complex concepts (Kloeppel & Hollins, 1989). Support groups in particular have been shown to be effective in assisting students with limited verbal and social skills (Berg, 1978) and are recommended for students as young as eleven years old (Hickey, 1993).

While providing opportunities to share information, teachers need to adopt procedures for value clarification. Teachers should handle religious concepts with care, assuring that they do not legislate their own beliefs. Educators also need to be aware of school policy and community views related to physical contact by a teacher and a student (i.e. touching and hugging) (Crenshaw, 1990).

As part of understanding values, children must develop strategies to cope with stress. Teachers must realize that children demonstrate a wide range of coping behaviors, including direct confrontation with death issues, detachment and complete avoidance. Educators should consider maintaining structure and routine so that the child has a sense of stability. Within that structure, teachers may explore creative ways for children to express grief. Suggestions include role playing (Dahlgren & Praeger-Decker, 1979; Crenshaw 1990), modeling, drawing and using puppets (Rucker, Thompson, & Dickerson, 1978). Some children will learn coping by participating in death rituals (Reeves & Knowles, 1981), remembering the person in a positive way (McDaniel, 1989), and setting as well as working toward personal goals.

Older students may also respond through self-expressive activities. Recommendations include keeping a journal where the student is encouraged to write expressions of grief, creating a scrapbook that contains memorabilia of the deceased, and sending a balloon filled with notes to the deceased in the air (Kandt, 1994). When follow-up is done with each of these activities the teacher has the opportunity to allow students to discuss their concerns. The most important variable in activities such as these is that it provides an opportunity for the teacher to listen to the grieving student (O'Brien, Goodenow, & Espin, 1991).

In addition to helping children cope, teachers need a means to help themselves, peers and other adults grieve (Tait & Ward, 1987; Keith & Ellis, 1978). Initially, they need to recognize the components of the grieving process and be aware that they may not, at that time, have the energy to help students grieve. Teachers must remember that each person grieves differently and should not be offended by a grieving person's behavior. It is important that people be allowed to display a variety of grieving behaviors such as crying (Tait & Ward, 1987). Additionally, teachers need to be willing to utilize the support systems available within the school and community. As with children, adults need coping skills such as remembering the person in a positive way, resuming routine, sharing feelings and keeping a professional perspective.

An important component to the grieving process is the involvement of the families and other members of the school community (Romanoff, 1993). It is important for the adults to have open communication lines (Snyder, 1993; Munsch, 1993; Chomicki, Sobsey, Sauvageot, & Wilgosh, 1995). This flow of communication may fulfill a dual purpose. Parents and the school personnel will understand how students are reacting during a time of grief and the adults will have a forum to discuss issues related to their feelings. As the adults assist children with developing a support group, they, in turn, will be generating a foundation for their own expression of grief.

Typically, teachers do not use counseling resources on a frequent basis and may be unfamiliar with the benefits associated with mental health personnel. When grieving is an issue there are local and national agencies that can help. Locally, teachers may contact either public or private mental health facilities. Many private agencies offer free crisis intervention counseling and/or short term care. Most social workers, counselors and psychologists are willing to consider a sliding fee for services. Clergy from the community are also an important assistance at this time. Teachers can also contact area hospice groups which frequently are associated with the local hospital. The local public and university libraries may also be centers for materials. Subject searches such as bereavement, death and grief may yield information about books for children and adults that can be borrowed. When researching topics related to death and grieving, teachers will discover that they have left educationally related journals and materials and entered the realm of mental health and counseling.

Nationally, there are several organizations that have materials about death and grieving. The Rainbow Connection [477 Hannah Branch Road, Burnsville, North Carolina 28714, phone (704) 675-9670, fax (704) 675-9687] offers *The Compassion Books Catalog* as a mail order services. In addition to training and workshops, audio tapes, video tapes and books are available for purchase. Resources are offered for children, adults and professionals; The Good Grief Program [Judge Baker Children's Center, 295 Longwood

Avenue, Boston, Massachusetts 02115, phone (671) 232-8390] has resources
and offers consultation to individuals who are grieving. The National Center for Death Education Library [Mount Ida College, 777 Deadham Street,
Newton Centre, Massachusetts 02159, (617) 969-7000, x249] has resources
about death and grieving.

SUMMARY

With the increased number of children with complex health concerns attending schools, death is becoming a more conspicuous part of a teacher's
repertoire of skills. Teachers must understand that students' ability to cope
with death and grief relates directly to the students' educational strengths
and weaknesses. As with any other aspect of a student's academic program,
educators must use their knowledge of the individual's developmental
progress, cognitive functioning, and social perception to assist in best explaining the grieving process. Likewise, educators must realize that an expression of grief is related to cultural, and social, variables. Variables such as
these change over time and are affected by the past interactions of the individuals involved with the deceased. Additionally, in order to provide appropriate intervention, teachers must be aware that all who grieve exhibit a wide
degree and intensity of symptoms when expressing grief.

Limited information about death and grief is currently available in the
educational literature. Few teacher training programs include discussion of
this topic as a part of their preparation programs. Given the changing face of
today's classrooms, institutions of higher education, practicing teachers and
school administrators must give serious consideration to this topic. Research
must learn more about how children, especially those with exceptionalities
grieve. Teachers need to become aware of the various symptoms of grief and
how to help students and colleagues deal with their response to death.
Schools and educational agencies must develop policies and crisis management plans as part of their responsibility to serve the members of the educational community. Death is often seen as the end. Yet, to the education
field offers the opportunity for new beginnings.

Epilogue

Sometimes when we hear the life stories of others we recognize how very lucky we have been. I have been lucky because there are people who believe that this work is important. During the writing of this book, Dr. Naomi Zigmond and I, through the University of Pittsburgh, were awarded a 3-year grant from the Office of Special Education Programs, U.S. Department of Education, Washington, DC. The grant supported the continuation and investigation of my research of children surviving childhood acute lymphoblastic leukemia with deleterious side effects in their educational careers and in their psychosocial interactions with others. The grant had been an enormous undertaking but once again, its qualitative nature had given us 27,000 pages of rich data to continue to bridge the gap between oncology and education, hospital, home, and school. We have, through this project, interviewed children newly diagnosed, children 5 years post treatment, adults who are long-term survivors of childhood ALL, as well as 32 teachers, school nurses, and principals who have received these children back into their schools and classrooms. I believe that the findings from the grant have helped pave the way for children who are stricken with a life-threatening illness to have the opportunity to lead a quality life.

Many of us go through life complaining about our problems or our lots in life instead of looking at life's greatest gifts. I believe we should not focus on the negative parts of living on this earth, but rather learn from our journeys, trials, and tribulations so we are able through ourselves to give life lessons as gifts back to others. To those who read this book, I hope you see it as a gift, just as it was a gift given to me to write it. I no longer look at my life in the same way. We often meet someone, go somewhere, or experience something that changes the course of our lives. In pursuit of the investigation of surviving childhood acute lymphoblastic leukemia, I have changed my thinking, my feeling, and my philosophy of life. What greater impact can one have than to have survivors teach you the true meaning of life? To all the individuals who have contributed to this research, we should be viewed as individuals who were truly lucky enough to be given the gift of this book to positively change the course of the lives of others as well as our own life.

Appendix 1

Bibliotherapy

Without memory, there is no healing.
Without forgiveness, there is no future.

—Archbishop Desmond Tutu

The Greeks and Romans were the first to use books as a form of interactive therapy between the reader and the use of literature. Definitions of *bibliotherapy* started to surface between the 1930s and the 1940s. The most simplified definition is "the use of books [or other media] to help understand problems and solve problems" (Bibliotherapy, 1993, p. 2). Bibliotherapy can cross many disciplines (library science, psychology, education, counseling, and medicine) in its attempt to use literature as a means of independent interaction with the reader over a life situation. However, it should be understood that the use of a bibliotherapy should not be an exclusive measure but should be viewed as an adjunct to other methods of counseling. Bibliotherapy can provide a system for individuals that offers a dual therapy approach that can enhance their ability to understand, accept, or solve their problems.

A bibliotherapy should be used when developing an individual's self-concept; enhancing an individual's understanding of human behavior; encouraging a person to be self-reflective; examining interests within the person; relieving emotional or mental pressure; lessening a person's anxiety about a problem by realizing other people have shared this problem as well; recognizing there is more than one way to solve a problem; developing an open discussion concerning the problem; supporting an individual in their plan to formulate a reasonable and active approach to solve the problem; and recognizing the possibility of more than one solution to a difficulty (Bibliotherapy, 1993, p. 2). *Bibliotherapy* means, in simple terms, "healing through books." I believe that a bibliotherapy can serve as a cathartic and insightful springboard, especially if there exists a sense of discomfort, fear, or lack of initial communication, providing stimulation in dealing with the issue of disclosure within a family, a classroom, with friends, or with the individual who has the difficulty in a free and open context to begin communication between individuals.

This bibliotherapy contains only literature that I felt had merit in dealing with the issue of children with cancer. The contents cover the forms of books, tapes, videos, and Internet sites for parents, children, families, psychologists, and teachers as related to survival. However, a few of the entries (for example, *Sadako* under "Children's Books") deal with the possibility of the death of a child and the coming to terms of this with a peaceful and dignified acceptance for children. I did provide my synopsis of each of the items listed in the bibliotherapy to help with an appropriate selection given the situation. However, I still recommend, whatever the choice is from this selection, that the individual preview it before using or recommending it in a given circumstance.

I hope this bibliotherapy, which was especially chosen and developed specifically for this book around the issue of children with life-threatening illnesses and more specifically cancer. I hope it will be of help and service to all those who have encountered and are dealing with the struggle of a child a serious illness or having to face the illness of someone else.

CHILDREN'S BOOKS

The Amazing Hannah, Look at Everything I Can Do!
by Amy Klett and Dave Klett
2003
Ages 1–5

A 28 page picture book written for a child who has been diagnosed with cancer. It has real-life photographs and it describes things related to the hospital—hospital stays, special friends, tests, treatment and germ care.

Beat the Turtle Drum
by Constance C. Greene
1976
Ages 10–14

A sensitive young girl comes to terms with the accidental death of her younger sister.

Blow Me a Kiss, Miss Lily
1990

When her best friend, an old lady named Miss Lily, passes away, Sara learns that the memory of a loved one never dies.

Bridge to Terabithia
By Katerine Paterson
1977
Ages 10–14

When Jess' new friend Leslie dies, Jess is confused and lonely until he decides to introduce another to Leslie's magic land of Terabithia.

Chemo, Craziness & Comfort, My Book About Childhood Cancer
by Nancy Keene and Trevor Romain
2003
Ages 6–12

A resource book that gives practical advice for children diagnosed with cancer. It has warm and funny illustrations and it is easy to read to the help child and parents make sense of cancer and its treatment.

Dear Bruno
by Alice Trillin
New Press; New York, NY, 1996.
ages: 10–up   grades: 5–up

In a letter to a young boy with cancer, a young female cancer survivor shares her experiences with the cancer "dragon." The author provides a delightful yet honest testimony to the childhood cancer experience. The whimsical illustrations capture the heart and soul.

The Fall of Freddie the Leaf
by Leo Buscaglia
Slack; Thorofare, NJ, 1992
ages: 4–8

This is a touching story about the acceptance and inevitability of dying. It is a beautifully written story of Freddie the Leaf as he takes his journey through the seasons of life. You will watch Freddie grow, thrive, and eventually decline in the fall. The author's sensitive treatment of the subject illustrates the balance between life and death.

Hang Tough, Paul Mather
by Alfred Slote
J. B. Lippincott; Philadelphia, PA, 1973.
ages: 10–14   grades: 5–8

This is a story of a 12-year-old Little League pitcher named Paul who learns that he has leukemia. Throughout the book, Paul has to deal with not only his illness, but the protectiveness of his parents and the knowledge that he may only have a short time left to play baseball. An understanding doctor helps Paul overcome his inner conflict and play out his short season with dignity, courage, and undaunted spirit.

Helen the Fish
by Nancy White Carlstrom and Virginia L. Kroll
1992

When six-year-old Hannah's beloved goldfish dies after a relatively long life, she seeks comfort from her older brother Seth.

Hospital Days, Treatment Ways: A Coloring Book
National Cancer Institute, Office of Cancer Communications, 1988.

NIH Publication No. 91-2085
Available at no cost from National Cancer Institute, Building 31, Room
10A24, Bethesda, MD 20892
ages: 4–7

This informative coloring book is designed to help parents and children
become familiar with the hospital routine, the tests, and the treatments
that they may undergo. The book contains illustrations with both brief and
more detailed descriptions of various medical treatments. It is important
that children review this book with parents so that they can adequately express their feelings and concerns. This book provides an opportunity to
discuss exactly what can be expected during treatment and can help the
family avoid unnecessary anxiety.

*I Want to Grow Hair, I Want to Grow Up, I Want to Go to Boise: Children Sur-
viving Cancer*
by Erma Bombeck
Harper & Row; New York, NY, 1989.
ages: 10–up   grades: 5–up

This heartwarming book brings us the stories of children surviving cancer.
Along the way, readers get to know the mothers, fathers, siblings, friends,
schoolmates, relatives, doctors, and teachers of these very optimistic and
insightful children. The children portrayed have every hope of beating the
odds and their stories should be read by everyone. After reading this book,
no one will remain the same.

I Will Sing Life: Voices from the Hole in the Wall Gang
by Larry Berger, Dahlia Lithwick, & Seven Campers
Little, Brown; Boston, MA, 1992.
ages: all

In this inspirational book, 7 campers from the Hole in the Wall Gang camp
for kids with life-threatening illnesses tell their stories. The campers share
their insights, laughter, hopes, and fears with the reader. The book includes inspirational poems written by the children. There is also an audio
version of this book.

Kathy's Hats: A Story of Hope
by Trudy Krisher
Albert Whitman; Morton Grove, IL, 1992.
ages: 5–10   grades: K–5

In this heartwarming book, a mother tells the story of her daughter Kathy's battle with cancer. Kathy's love of hats comes in handy when the chemotherapy treatments she receives for her cancer make her hair fall out. The words and illustrations depict the emotions involved in dealing with cancer and the embarrassment felt when hair is lost. This book could be read in the classroom to encourage a discussion and to sensitize children to the cancer experience.

The Kids Book About Death and Dying by and for Kids
by E. E. Rofers
1985
Ages 4-8

Fourteen children offer facts and advice to give young readers a better understanding of death.

Living with Cancer
by Dr. Simon Smail
Franklin Watts; New York, NY, 1990.
ages: 10–12   grades: 5–6

This book provides basic information and colorful illustrations related to cancer. Topics discussed include how the body works, symptoms and warning signs of cancer, the necessary tests associated with diagnosing cancer, forms of treatment, and possible precautionary measures to prevent cancer. It is an appropriate reference for teachers or parents who will need to discuss relevant issues with children.

May I Cross Your Golden River
by Page Dixon
1986

An 18-year-old boy tries to cope with the realization that he has a fatal disease.

My Book for Kids With Cansur: A Child's Autobiography of Hope
by Jason Gaes
Melius & Peterson; Aberdeen, SD, 1987.
ages: 5–8   grades: 1–3   32 pp.

Written when the author was 7, this book describes Jason Gaes's successful battle with cancer. The text of the book is in Jason's own handwriting, complete with his own style and second-grade spelling. He describes being diagnosed with cancer, the side effects of the treatments, and his fears. This is a useful book for a classroom setting. The young author reaches out to the child reader in a truthful yet charming manner. His descriptions, along with his brothers' illustrations, provide a forum for questions and discussions.

Rosey in the Present Tense
by Louise Hawes
1999

Unable to accept the sudden death of his Japanese American girlfriend, Rose, 17-year-old Franklin finds that she has come back to him as a spirit and eventually realizes that he must let her go.

Sadako
by Eleanor Coerr & Ed Young
G. P. Putnam's Sons; New York, NY, 1993.
ages: 7–12   grades: 2–6

The writing of this book is very descriptive in nature, pulling the reader in, revealing a touching drama of childhood cancer. Sadako, the young Japanese girl depicted in the story, developed leukemia as a result of the atomic bomb dropped on Hiroshima. Readers are taken on a journey with Sadako and learn about her feelings surrounding the illness, her courageous fight, and eventually the peaceful acceptance of her own death.

Snowdrops for Cousin Ruth
by Susan Katz
1998

Nine-year-old Johanna and eighty-two year-old Cousin Ruth try to help their family heal after the accidental death of Johanna's younger brother.

What Happened When Grandma Died
by Peggy Barker
1984
Ages 3–8

On the way to her grandma's funeral a little girl asks her dad what happens when people die. Her dad explains that there are things that get left behind when someone dies, but that God promises three new things— a new body, a new home in heaven, and a new life with God.

What's Heaven?
by Maria Shriver
1999

Borne from actual questions by her own daughters, journalist Maria Shiver's book is a gentle narrative following conversations that pass between a mother and a young daughter in the days immediately following the death of the child's special grandmother.

When Dinosaurs Die: A Guide to Understanding Death
by Laurene Krasny Brown
1996
Ages 4–8

Presents a balanced, comprehensive and age appropriate explanation of why death occurs and other such issues, and suggest sensible, specific tactics for coping with the resulting loneliness, fright and anger.

Who is Ben?
by Charlotte Zolotow
1997

On a moonless, starless night, a young boy feels at one with the darkness, thinking about where he came from before he was born and where will he go after he dies.

VIDEOS

The videos listed are available to borrow or purchase through
Candlelighters Childhood Cancer Foundation Canada
55 Eglinton Avenue East, Suite 401
Toronto, Ontario M4P 1G8
Phone: (416) 489-6440
http://www.candlelighters.ca/

Aarvy Aardvark Finds Hope
(Rainbow Connection, 1994, 45 mins.)

Adventures of Rufus and Andy: The Rescue
(Magic Lantern Communications, 1991, 15 mins.)

Childhood Cancer: Siblings Speak Out
(Produced by Children's Hospital of Denver, 22 mins.)

Childhood Leukaemia
(Canadian Learning, 60 mins.)

Children in Pain: An Overview
(Magic Lantern Communications, 1992, 27 mins.)

Day by Day
(G. Curtis, CTRS Film Production, 40 mins.)

*Dr. Elisabeth Kubler-Ross Interviews Childhood Cancer Patients and
Their Families*
(Elisabeth Kubler-Ross Center, 60 mins.)

Draw Me a Song
(National Film Board, 1990, 8 mins.)

Growing Up with Cancer
(Midland Video Production)

Hair Loss
(Magic Lantern Communications, 1987, 12 mins.)

Healing Spirit
(National Film Board, 1992, 57 mins.)

I Had a Dream
(Profile Communication and the Canadian Cancer Society, 29 mins.)

I'm Still Me
(Susan Linn, 18 mins.)

Just Kids
(National Film Board, 1993, 27 mins.)

Kids and Cancer
(CBC Health Show, 1995, 12 mins.)

Mister Rogers Talks About Childhood Cancer
(*Mister Rogers' Neighborhood* and the American Cancer Society, 1989, 26 mins.)

Mister Rogers Talks with Parents About Childhood Cancer
(*Mister Rogers' Neighborhood* and the American Cancer Society, 1989, 25 mins.)

My Hair's Falling Out . . . Am I Still Pretty?
(New Generation Pictures, 1992)

No Greater Gift
(Magic Lantern Communications, 1986, 30 mins.)

No Tears . . . No Fears: Children with Cancer Coping with Pain
(Leora Kuttner, Multimedia Productions and Canadian Cancer Society, BC/Yukon Division, 1986, 28 mins.)

Not Just a Cancer Patient
(Canadian Learning, 23 mins.)

One, Two, Three . . . Ouchless!
(Funded by Candlelighters Childhood Cancer Foundation Canada, Astra Pharma, and The Hospital for Sick Children, Toronto, 1993, 7 mins.)

Pediatrics: Leukaemia and Other Childhood Cancers
(Canadian Learning, 20 mins.)

Princes in Exile
(National Film Board, Canada, 1990, 101 mins.)

Sherri (originally It's a Privilege to Know You)
(Prisma-light, Toronto, 1995, 22 mins.)

Special Love
(Modern Talking Pictures Service)

Treating Children with Cancer
(Canadian Learning, 55 mins.)

What Do I Tell my Children?
(Aquarius Productions, 30 mins.)

When a Child has Cancer
(American Cancer Society, 23 mins.)

Why, Charlie Brown, Why?
(Charles Schultz Video)

INTERNET SITES FOR CHILDREN

http://cancernet.nci.nih.gov/occdocs/KidsHome.html: The KidsHome page, sponsored by the National Cancer Institute, contains literature, games, activities, and stories for kids with cancer and their families. Also included are many links to other fun and informative Web sites for kids.

http://funrsc.fairfield.edu/jfleitas/contents.html: The intent of this site is to sensitize children to the experience of growing up with a serious medical condition. Contributions, ideas, and suggestions made by children with medical problems are included throughout this site. The homepage contains links to stories, poems, and activities for children.

http://funrsc.fairfield.edu/jfleitas/contents.html: Bandaids and Blackboards is an excellent site for youngsters with chronic or serious illness. This site offers practical suggestions for helping young children, their parents, and their educators to cope with the many issues surrounding surviving chronic illness especially those involving school reentry.

http://starbright.org/project/world/index.html: Starbright is a new, revolutionary, and award-winning site for hospitalized children with serious illness. The ultimate goal is improving the quality of life of seriously ill children. The site essentially acts as a network play space; a playground that links ill children regardless of location and capability.

http://www.ability.ns.ca/young.html: This site contains artwork, articles, and stories submitted by kids and teens. Users can submit their own work to the site through e-mail. There are also links to other sites for kids.

http://minuteman.com/specialove/: Special Love offers year-round programs and provides kids with cancer and their families the opportunity to enjoy normal activities through camps, trips, and weekend outings. This site offers families a network of support. Survivors share their personal trials and triumphs in fighting this disease.

http://www.monkey-boy.com/melinda/: This page was created by a young girl with cancer and her father. Melinda's wish was to create this page for other kids with cancer and their families. Her site is full of information, fun stories, and activities. It also includes links to communicate with other "Cancer Kids."

http://oncolink.upenn.edu/resources/kids/index.html: OncoLink's Kid's Corner contains resources for children with cancer and their families. There are a variety of links to information and activities as well as links to communicate with other cancer kids.

INTERNET SITES FOR PARENTS

http://cancer.med.upenn.edu/: OncoLink, sponsored by the University of Pennsylvania Cancer Center, is a resource providing detailed information on specific cancers and the results of recent research conducted.

http://cancernet.nci.nih.gov/: CancerNet, a comprehensive site, provides links to cancer information for the public, health professionals, and basic researchers.

http://minuteman.com/specialove/: Special Love offers year-round programs and provides kids with cancer and their families the opportunity to enjoy normal activities through camps, trips, and weekend outings. This site offers the family a network of support. Survivors share their personal trials and triumphs in fighting this disease.

http://mypage.ihost.com/CCC/index.html: The Children's Cancer Center is an organization dedicated to providing children with cancer and their families with the emotional, financial, and educational support necessary to coping with the illness. The center provides a variety of services.

htpp://www.candlelighters.org/: This national organization primarily offers support to children with childhood cancer and their families. It serves as an information network dedicated to enhancing the quality of life of children and teens with cancer, their families, and all who care for and about them. This site offers the family a multitude of services: parent support groups, parent-to-parent visitations, summer camps, and information on childhood cancer and treatment, and sponsors conferences at both the regional and the national levels.

http://www.candlelighters.ca/bursary.html: The Candlelighters Childhood Cancer Foundation offers college scholarships for survivors of childhood cancer.

http://www.candlelighters.ca/tochthesky.html: This site offers a unique program to develop coping skills in children living with life-threatening illness. The Touch the Sky Program encourages parents and children to work together in the healing process.

http://www.interlog.com/~fcc/: Families of Children with Cancer is an organization devoted to the education, support, and advocacy for families living with effects of childhood cancer. Includes many links to more information.

http://www.kidswithcancer.com/c/cancer/: Kids with Cancer is a page created by parents whose kids have been diagnosed with some form of childhood cancer. Their mission is to provide accurate information, resources, support, and links to reliable sources of information for other parents of childhood cancer patients.

http://www.nccf.org/: The National Childhood Cancer Foundation's site offers facts on childhood cancer as well as inspiring stories and links to other information sources.

http://www.squirreltales.com/index.htm: The Never-Ending Squirrel Tale Web site was created by a parent of a child diagnosed with cancer. This mother has gathered practical tips and encouraging stories. She also welcomes you to share your stories on her site.

GENERAL INFORMATION

Afraid to Ask: A Book for Families to Share About Cancer
by Judylaine Fine
Lothrop, Lee, & Shepard Books; New York, NY, 1986.

This book, written for adolescents and adults, provides down-to-earth explanations of what cancer is, who gets cancer, and the possible prevention of cancer. Through interviews with professionals, patients, and their family members, the author gives the answers that young people will need to understand the biology of the disease and the emotional problems it entails. This book also discusses the different types of cancer and the treatments involved.

Answers to 25 Questions You Were Always Afraid to Ask
by Errol C. Friedberg, MD
Freeman; New York, NY, 1992.

This informative guide gives non-technical answers to the questions commonly asked by cancer patients and their families. The information is clearly written and organized so that a cancer patient can be equipped to cope with the illness.

Back to School: A Handbook for Educators of Children with Life-Threatening Diseases in the Yeshiva/Day School System
Chai Lifeline, 1995

To receive a copy, write to 48 West 25th St., New York, NY 10010 or call (212) 465-1300. Comprehensive topics include diagnosis, planning school re-entry, infection control in schools, needs of junior and senior high students, children with special educational needs, and saying good-bye when a child dies. Bibliography and resource list.

Back to School: A Handbook for Parents of Children with Cancer
American Cancer Society.

For a free copy call (800) ACS-1234. Booklet provides information on school reentry, classroom presentations, advocacy, legal issues, and special needs.

Bereavement and Children
by Alan D. Wolfelt, Ph.D.

He is a clinical thanatologist and director of the Center for Loss and Life Transition, an organization dedicated to furthering our understanding of the complex set of the emotion we call grief." He also gives educational seminars. He has written several books including: *Sarah's Journey, Healing the Bereaved Child*, and *A Child's View of Grief*. Dr. Wolfelt has also written numerous articles including "Ten Common Myths about Children and Grief," "Left and Left Out: Teaching Children to Grieve through a Rehabilitation Curriculum," "Grief Gardening: Ages and Stages," "Helping Grieving Children at School," "Helping Classrooms Cope with Traumatic Events," and "ADHD and the Bereaved Child." Videotapes are also available: *A Child's View of Grief, A Teen's View of Grief*, and *Training Videos on Grief*. You can receive an order form for materials and you can get back issues of up to 5 years of *Bereavement Magazine* that contain some of Dr. Wolfelt's work from Bereavement Publishing, Inc., 8133 Telegraph Drive, Colorado Springs, CO 80920, phone: (719) 282-1948; Fax: (719) 282-1850. You can request for free: Companion Press Publication Catalog, Center for Loss Educational Seminars Catalog, and Centerpiece Newsletter; Phone: (970) 226-6050; Fax: (970) 226-6051; Email: wolfelt@centerforloss.com; Web site: www.centerforloss.com.

Bereavement Publishing
5125 North Union Blvd., Suite #4
Colorado Springs, CO 80918
Phone: (719) 266-0006
Fax: (719) 266-0012 or (888) 60-4-HOPE (4673)
Email: griefmag@aol.com

Provides a product catalog filled with books, booklets, cards, cassette tapes, and so forth. Also, publishes a magazine.

Bobby's Books,

"Bobby's Books is a collection of children's literature that provides families with information and a choice of books to use with children as they discuss grief, change, and loss. This project is funded by community donations, the Barbara Bush Foundation for Family Literacy, and the New York Life Foundation/Literacy Volunteers of America." This organization has books on AIDS, cancer, suicide, death and dying, aging, illness and death of a sibling, disabilities and coping, the Oklahoma City bombing, coping with hospitalizations, to name some. The books from this organization are books for children of all ages. Interestingly, they do have a list of children's books and summaries of each book specifically for the middle school student. Request information from Columbus Public Schools, Department of Community Education, North Education Center, 100 Arcadia Avenue, Columbus, OH 43202; Phone: (614) 365-5146; Fax: (614) 365-5239; Email: Pkrenzke@aol.com

A Cancer Survivor's Almanac: Charting Your Journey
Barbara Hoffman (Ed.)
Chronimed; Minneapolis, MN, 1996.

This book, written by the survivors and professionals who founded the cancer survivorship movement, will serve as a guide to help survivors, caregivers, families, and friends plan for the survivorship journey. It provides helpful information and necessary support that will improve the quality of life for cancer survivors. Topics discussed in detail include taking care of medical, emotional, social, and financial needs. This all-encompassing guide clearly addresses the many issues in coping with the cancer experience.

Chicken Soup for the Surviving Soul
by Jack Canfield, Mark Victor Hansen, Patty Aubery, & Nancy Mitchell, RN
Health Communications; Deerfield Beach, FL, 1996.

This book contains 101 inspiring stories of cancer survivors that will encourage you to be hopeful, persuade you to reach out for and accept support, and invite you to share your feelings. Through the experiences of others, this book will help you through times of frustration, challenge, pain, and suffering. Throughout the book, you will be introduced to many cancer patients who offer support through their understanding of the cancer experience.

Childhood Cancer Survivors: A Guide to the Future
Nancy Keene, Wendy Hobbie, & Kathy Ruccione
O'Reilly & Associates; Sebastopol, CA, 2000.

Deals with the late effects of treatment for childhood cancer. Includes stories from childhood cancer survivors, emotional issues, insurance, jobs, relationships, and how to be healthy.

Childhood Leukemia: A Guide for Families, Friends, and Caregivers.
by Nancy Keene & Honna Janes-Hodder
O'Reilly & Associates; 3rd ed., 1999

This is a very well-written and comprehensive book on childhood leukemia. It is easy to read and it has a lot of information. Honna Janes-Hodder and Nancy Keene, the authors, each had a child who had been diagnosed with childhood leukemia. They use excerpts from parents throughout the book to make it not just an informational book but a book that also has a human element. Some of the chapters include What is Leukemia?; About Acute Lymphoblastic Leukemia (ALL); Signs and Symptoms; Parents' Responses to Diagnosis; Chemotherapy-Related Hair Loss and Nausea; After Treatment; Regaining Normalcy. The book also provides an immense listing of resources and organizations that can be helpful to the cancer patient, their family, and friends. You can order the book by calling 1-800-998-9938. Also, you can visit the Web site http://patientcenters.com.ChildhoodLeukemia-Centers. By visiting this Web site, you are able to read and/or print out some of the chapters to the book.

Children with Cancer: A Comprehensive Reference Guide for Parents
by Jeanne Munn Bracken
Oxford University Press; New York, NY, 1986

This resource book is practical and useful for parents and professionals who need to quickly gain an understanding of the many issues that arise when a child is diagnosed with cancer. As a resource librarian and parent of a child who has survived cancer, the author provides honest, warm, and supportive insights for coping in addition to comprehensive references and listings of organizations and treatment centers for searching out the best care available across the country.

Children with Cancer: A Comprehensive Reference Guide for Parents
by Jeanne Munn Bracken

A wealth of information essential to help a child or family through this ordeal. From sophisticated, hard-to-find medical facts to tips on handling side effects. 407 pp.; Hardcover :$37.50; Softcover :$13.45.

Death and the Classroom: A Teacher's Guide to Assist Grieving Students
by Kathleen Cassini and Jacqueline Rogers

Chapters address teacher reactions and comments; students' concept of death; directives from teacher as they interact with students and family on the first and second day following death; terminology defining and explaining visitation, funeral services, and cemetery proceedings, spontaneous memorial service, and planned memorial service; normal and abnormal grief reactions; national resource lists and media suggestions; needs of teachers and school staff; and long-term support for the grieving student. 108 pp.; $17.95 + $2.50 S/H.Griefwork of Cincinnati, Inc. 1445 Colonial Drive, Suite A, Cincinnati, OH 45238-3839, Phone: (513) 922-1202, Fax: (513) 922-8285, Online: griefmag@aol.com

Diagnosis Cancer
by Wendy Schlessel Harpham, MD
Norton; London, 1992.

Written by a physician who is a cancer survivor, this book provides insight into the cancer experience from the perspective of the patient as well as the physician. The author addresses topics such as prognosis, treatment, pain relief, and remission. This book offers patients and their family members a crash course in navigating the critical first months of cancer management.

. . . The Diagnosis is Cancer . . . : A Psychological and Legal Resource Handbook for Cancer Patients, Their Families, and Helping Professionals
by Edward J. Larschan, JD, PhD, with Richard J. Larschan, PhD
Bull Publishing; Palo Alto, CA, 1986

This resource handbook addresses the emotional impact and legal implications of acquiring and living with a life-threatening illness. The author, a cancer survivor himself, shares his expertise as a psychologist and attorney. Beyond his own personal experience, the author reveals the importance of taking action to enhance one's emotional and financial well-being.

Drying Their Tears
Produced by CART, Communications Division,
Markham University, P.O. Box 55050, Little Rock, AR 72215
or call (800) 482-8561 or (501) 660-7614.

Very well done video and it is intended to help counselors, teachers, and other professionals help children with grief, anger, and fear. There are three parts to this video: training facilitators, and a part for children ages 5–8 and ages 9–teens.

Educating the Child with Cancer
by Patricia Deasy-Spinetta and Elisabeth Irvin
Candlelighters Childhood Cancer Foundation and Kensington, MD: 2003

For a free copy call (800) 366-CCCF. The book chapters cover educational issues, peer relationships, school reentry, liaison programs, classroom presentations, cognitive late effects, preparing for college, college alternatives, legal issues, and siblings.

Everyone's Guide to Cancer Therapy
by Malin Dollinger, MD, Ernest Rosenbaum, MD, & Greg Cable
Andrews & McMeel; Kansas City, MO, 1991.

This extremely well-organized reference book offers an excellent step-by-step approach to the process of understanding cancer and the kinds of treatment involved. The book explains the basis for the many tests all cancer patients must undergo. It explains clearly and simply what to expect from various forms of therapy. The authors also suggest many ways that individuals can cope and contribute to their own well-being during recovery.

For the Love of Teddi: The Story Behind Camp Good Days and Special Times
by Lou Buttino
Praeger, New York, 1990

This book shows how a family tried to make something positive out of the devastation of childhood cancer. For the love of Teddi is a real life drama—an American love story. But most of all it is an inspiration of how something good and enduring can come from an experience as uniquely tragic as the death of a child. 198 pp.; Hardcover: $24.95; Soft-cover: $14.50.

From Victim to Victor: For Cancer Patients and Their Families
by Harold H. Benjamin, PhD
Dell Publishing; New York, NY, 1987.

In this book, Dr. Benjamin speaks out frankly to answer questions about cancer and the emotional aspects involved. He offers scientific evidence to support the beneficial effects of positive emotions. This book also suggests specific techniques to help the cancer patient emotionally, psychologically, and physically. Topics discussed include cancer and its causes, disclosure, and dealing with reactions to cancer.

Grief Comes to Class: A Teacher's Guide
by Majel Gliko-Braden
Centering Corp. Omaha

To receive a copy, write Centering Corporation, 1531 N. Saddle Creek Rd., Omaha, NE 68104 or call (402) 553-1200. Chapters cover grief responses, the bereaved student, teen grief, developmental stages, sample letter to parents, sample teacher/parent conference and the do's and don'ts.

Grief Support on the World Wide Web
An Internet Hotlist on Grief Support on the World Wide Web
Created by Patricia L. Frost, Lahore American School
http://www.kn.pacebell.com/wired/fil/pages/listgriefsupp.html

"This website is for those who are mourning the loss of a loved one. It is also for those people who want to help a grieving friend or family member." Topics include ideas to help people in mourning, children and teen grief, men and women grief, tributes and memorials to loved ones, and healing and grief resources.

Hairballs on My Pillow

To receive a copy, write CARTI, P.O. Box 55050, Little Rock, AR 72215 or call (800) 482-8561 or (501) 664-8573

$35.00 for video of interviews of children with cancer and their friends/ friendships. Newsletters for students, exercises and activities for students, information for the teacher related to cancer and school reentry for a child who has cancer.

Healing the Bereaved Child
by Dr. Alan Wolfelt
Fort Collins, CO, Companion Press, 1996

Excellent book on how a grieving child thinks, feels, and mourns. Some highlighted chapters include Helping the Grieving Adolescent, Counseling Techniques, Helping Children at School. Order online: griefmag@ aol.com.

Last Week My Brother Anthony Died
by Martha Hickman
Abingdon, TN, 1984

A preschooler shares her feelings when her infant brother dies. Very heartwarming book especially when a minister compares feelings to clouds as always there but always changing.

Lifetimes: A Beautiful Way to Explain Death to Children
by Bryan Mellonie
1983

Death is explained through the cycles of nature.

Mr. Rogers Talks About Childhood Cancer.
1990. Two videotapes, guidebook, and storybook.
45 minutes in length. VHS.
Call the American Cancer Society (800) ACS-2345.

Mr. Rogers in these videos talks to children about sharing their feelings with someone and he uses the characters from his television show (Land of Make Believe) to help him.

Mr. Rogers Talks with Parents About Childhood Cancer
Two videotapes, guidebook, pamphlet.
Video is 47 min. VHS.
Call the American Cancer Society (800) ACS-2345.

Tape one has interview with parents about how to handle emotions during the initial stages of treatment. Tape has sensitive interviews with bereaved parents.

One Day At A Time: Children Living with Leukemia
by Thomas Bergman
Gareth Stevens Children's Books; Milwaukee, WI, 1989.

In this book, the reader follows the dramatic stories of two young children, 2-year-old Hanna and 3-year-old Frederick who are being treated for childhood leukemia. Hanna has just begun her treatment and Frederick has been ill for approximately six months. Guided by these children, their parents, and their doctors, the reader takes a journey into the world of the leukemia patient. These pages not only contain insightful text but remarkable black-and-white photographs.

Project D.O.C.C. (Delivery of Chronic Care), School-Health-Parent Task Force, and the Parent Advocacy Group
Information can be obtained by contacting:
Patricia Weiner (one of the founders of D.O.C.C. and Medical Liaison),

Director of Child Life and Education Services,
Department of Pediatrics, North Shore University Hospital,
300 Community Drive, Manhasset, NY 11030
(516) 562-2567

A parent-directed pediatric residency training program at 11 hospitals throughout the United States. It has been implemented to keep the lines of communication open between families, school staff, and health care professionals. These services are important in the education of children with special health care needs.

The Psychosocial Dimensions of Cancer: A Practical Guide for Health Care Providers
by Richard Goldberg, MD & Robert M. Tull, PhD
Free Press/Macmillan; New York, NY, 1983

Although this text is intended for health care professionals, families will find it a great resource for providing emotional support to those living with cancer. Specifically, the author shares practical information for dealing with the child, the adolescent, and the adult with cancer. The goal of this book is to provide health care professionals and caregivers a better understanding of the total cancer experience.

Sam Fights Back
Leukemia Society of America
For a free copy call (800) 955-4LSA.

A coloring and activity book for 3–6 year old leukemia patients to learn about leukemia and how to deal with their feelings.

School Re-entry Resource Manual
Candlelighters Childhood Cancer Foundation, Toronto, 1992

For a copy write: CCCFC, 10 Alcorn Ave., Suite 200, Toronto, Ontario M4V 3B1 or call (416) 489-6440. This manual covers information for parents, educators, health care professionals on the topics of siblings, adolescence, survivor's quality of life, programs, bereavement, and grief.

Standing Together Standing Strong (video)
Dialogue Systems and Cancer Cured Kids, 1997
Approximate length: 40 min.

This video is the only one of its kind on the current market. It is a comprehensive video that includes dialogue from a news reporter, pediatric oncologists, hospital educator and nurse, teachers who have had children with cancer in their classrooms, parents of children who have cancer, children who have or had cancer, and a long-term survivor of childhood cancer. This exceptional video gives factual information about the disease of childhood leukemia with recommendations to parents, teachers, homebound tutors, other school personnel, school nurses, and guidance counselors who are all an important and essential part of a child's life during the duration of diagnosis, treatment, and cure. Information contained in this video is up-to-date and easily understood for both the layperson and the professional. If you are looking for a quick and accessible form of information on the subject of children with cancer as it relates to their school experiences, this video is a must "see and hear" video. Contact: Cancer Cured Kids, c/o Jamie Reish, President and Co-founder, P.O. Box 189, Old Westbury, NY 11568, Telephone: 516-484-8160.

Students with Cancer: A Resource for the Educator
U.S Department of Health and Human Services, 1987.
NIH Publication No. 91-2086
Available at no cost from National Cancer Institute, Building 31, Room 10A24, Bethesda, MD 20892.

This booklet has been developed to help answer some of the questions that teachers of students with cancer may have. General explanations of the illness, treatments, and side effects are included. Suggested approaches for dealing with the student with cancer, his or her classmates and parents, serve as a useful resource for the educator. References to additional materials and organizations are also provided.

Talking with Your Child About Cancer
U.S. Department of Health and Human Services, 1990.
NIH Publication No. 91-2761

Available at no cost from National Cancer Institute, Building 31, Room 10A24, Bethesda, MD 20892.

This booklet provides detailed information on how to disclose to your child that he has cancer. The booklet describes the general stages in child development and what children tend to understand about a serious illness at different ages. Since children are naturally curious and your child knows and trusts you, he will expect you to answer most of his questions. This booklet offers some practical ideas to help you reassure your child during diagnosis and treatment and answer some of the questions he is likely to ask.

When Your Brother or Sister has Cancer
American Cancer Society
For a free copy call (800) ACS-2345.

This is a small booklet that helps to describe the feelings felt by siblings of a child who has cancer.

Why, Charlie Brown, Why?
by Charles M. Schultz
Topper Books, New Yor, 1990

A story about what happens when a friend becomes very ill. A true reflection of the encouraging story of childhood leukemia, complete with illustrations. Also in video. 58 pp.; Softcover: $10.45. Call the Leukemia Society of America at (800) 955-4LSA.

You Don't Have to Suffer: A Complete Guide to Relieving Cancer Pain for Patients and Their Families
by Susan S. Lang & Richard Patt, MD
Oxford University Press; New York, NY, 1994.

This is a resource book on cancer and the physical and emotional pain involved. The book explores all the pain-relieving options available, providing information on the major painkillers used in treatment and their side effects. Other topics discussed include mind-body approaches to easing pain and dealing with feelings of anxiety, denial, fear, isolation, guilt, anger, hopelessness.

Young People with Cancer: A Handbook for Parents
U.S. Department of Health and Human Services, 1991.
NIH Publication No. 92-2378
Available at no cost from National Cancer Institute, Building 31, Room 10A24, Bethesda, MD 20892.

This handbook combines medical information with practical suggestions for families of young cancer patients. This book can be viewed as a general guide toward what to expect and how to deal with childhood cancer. Topics discussed include the types of cancer, treatment procedures, and side effects, and tips for clinic visits and medical procedures. Special consideration is given to the emotional impact of cancer on patients and family members.

Your Child in the Hospital: A Practical Guide for Parents
by Nancy Keene
O'Reilly & Associates; Sebastopol, CA: rev. ed. 1999.

A great small guide that has parent stories that will help parents prepare a child on what to expect at the hospital physically and emotionally.

Appendix 2

Glossary of Medical Terms

acute lymphoblastic leukemia (ALL).   Usually a disease of children. Features not fully formed white blood cells that collect in the bone marrow, blood, lymph nodes, spleen, liver, and other organs. The number of normal blood cells is reduced. Also known as acute lymphocytic leukemia.

acute myeloid leukemia (AML).   An acute form of leukemia characterized by a massive proliferation of mature and immature abnormal granulocytes. There are seven different types of AML.

acute nonlymphoblastic leukemia (ANLL).   A form of acute leukemia. It is one-fourth as common as ALL. It usually attacks the white cells in the bone marrow that are not lymphoblasts, but still has similar symptoms of ALL. Usually occurs in adolescence.

adenopathy.   A growth on any gland; especially a lymph gland.

adjuvant therapy.   Additional drug to another treatment designed to enhance the effectiveness of the primary treatment.

allogeneic bone marrow transplant.   Transplant in which bone marrow or stem cells from a donor, rather than the patient's own marrow, is infused.

alopecia.   Hair loss.

anemia.   Too few red blood cells in the bloodstream, resulting in insufficient oxygen to tissues and organs.

antibiotic.   A drug used to fight bacterial infections.

apheresis.   The peripheral blood stem cell collection process in which blood is taken from a patient and circulated through a machine that separates out stem cells. The remaining cells are returned to the patient.

aplasia. A failure to develop or form. In bone marrow aplasia, the marrow cavity is empty.

ataxia. Loss of balance.

autograft. Bone marrow removed from the patient to be used in an autologous bone marrow transplant.

autologous bone marrow transplant. Transplant in which the patient's own bone marrow, rather than the marrow from a donor, is infused during transplant to provide the body with a source of stem cells.

axillary node. One of the lymph glands of the armpit that help fight infections in the chest, armpit, neck, and arm.

bacteria. Microscopic organisms that invade human cells, multiply rapidly, and produce toxins that interfere with normal cell function.

B cells. Type of lymphocyte (white blood cell) that helps produce antibodies that destroy foreign substances.

biopsy. Removal of tissue for examination under a microscope, sometimes required to enable the doctor to make a proper diagnosis.

blast cell crisis. Patients with chronic myelogenous leukemia, the progression of the diseases to an "acute" advanced stage, evidenced by an increased number of immature white blood cells in the circulating blood. Sometimes loosely used to describe a rapid increase in the white blood cells count of any leukemic patient.

blast cells. Immature cells.

blood-brain barrier. Blood vessels located around the central nervous system with very closely spaced cells that make it difficult for potentially toxic substances—including anticancer drugs—to enter the brain and spinal cord.

blood type. Identification of proteins in a person's blood cells so that transfusions can be given with compatible blood products. Blood types are A+, A−, B+, B−, AB+, AB−, O+, O−.

bone marrow. Spongy tissue in the cavities of large bones, where the body's blood cells are produced.

bone marrow aspiration (biopsy). Procedure used to remove a sample of bone marrow, usually from the rear hipbone, for examination under the microscope.

bone marrow transplant (BMT). A procedure in which doctors replace bone marrow/stem cells that have been destroyed by high doses of chemotherapy and/or radiation.

cancer. Abnormal cells divide without control.

carcinogen. A substance or agent that produces cancer.

catheter.   Small, flexible plastic tube inserted into a portion of the body to remove fluids.

CBC (complete blood count).   Determines whether the proper number of red and white blood cells and platelets are present in the patient's blood.

central nervous system (CNS).   The body system that is made up of the brain, spinal cord, and nerves. The central nervous system is a natural sanctuary site for some leukemic cells and must be treated with chemotherapy and radiation.

central venous catheter.   Small, flexible plastic tube inserted into a large vein above the heart, through which drugs and blood products can be given, and blood samples withdrawn painlessly. Also called central line and Hickman catheter.

cerebrospinal fluid.   Fluid that surrounds and bathes the brain and spinal cord and provides a cushion from shocks.

cervical.   Referring to the neck or neckline.

chemotherapy.   Drug or combination of drugs designed to kill cancerous cells. It involves up to 30 drugs or combination of drugs used to destroy or block leukemic cells.

Children's Cancer Group.   An organization that designs and monitors pediatric clinical trials.

chronic.   Persisting for a long time.

Chronic myelogenous leukemia.   A disease that progresses slowly and is characterized by a proliferation of granulocyctes in the bone marrow. Usually associated with the Philadelphia chromosome.

clinical trial.   A study of the effectiveness of a drug or treatment.

colony stimulating factor.   Proteins that stimulate the production and growth of certain types of blood cells.

conjunctivitis.   Eye inflammation.

consolidation therapy.   A part of the protocol that consists of new combinations of drugs to destroy any cancer cells that survived induction.

contracture.   Shortening of muscle, skin, and other soft tissue, usually in the limbs. May occur in patients with chronic graft-versus-host disease.

cranial irradiation.   Exposure to heat, light, or x-ray that destroys cells that are cancerous to the entire skull area.   Side effects: loss of hair, headaches, dizziness, confusion, tiredness, memory difficulties.

cryopreservation.   To preserve by freezing. Bone marrow harvested for an autologous BMT, for example, is cryopreserved.

CT scan.   A three-dimensional x-ray. Also called a CAT scan or CT X-ray.

cytomegalovirus. A virus that lies dormant in many persons' bodies and frequently causes infection posttransplant.

cytoxan (cyclophosphamide). A drug used to treat many cancers and to prevent rejection in organ transplants. Blocks the growth of cells in the body. Used only a short time because this drug can cause cancer. It is important to drink a lot of fluids to help prevent kidney and bladder problems. Side effects: blood in urine, painful urination, dizziness, confusion, agitation, fever, chills, sore throat, tiredness, cough, joint pain, shortness of breath, missed menstrual periods, swelling in the feet or lower legs, unusual bleeding or bruising, unusually fast heartbeat, black, tarry stools, sores in mouth and on lips, frequent urination, unusual thirst, yellow eyes and skin, darkening of skin and fingernails, loss of hair, nausea or vomiting. Also known as cyclophosphamide.

dermatitis. A skin rash.

dysplasia. Alteration in the size, shape, and organization of cells or tissues.

edema. Abnormal accumulation of fluid.

electrolyte. Minerals found in the blood such as sodium potassium that must be maintained within a certain range to prevent organ malfunction.

encephalopathy. Abnormal functioning of the brain.

endocrine system. Secretes hormones into the bloodstream. Glands include thyroid, pituitary, pancreas, adrenal, and the gonads.

engraftment. When bone marrow infused during a BMT "takes" or is accepted by the patient, and begins producing blood cells.

enzyme. A protein that is capable of facilitating a chemical reaction.

eosinophil. A type of white blood cell that protects against infection.

fungus. A primitive life form that can cause infection in the body. Fungi that sometimes cause posttreatment infections are the *Candida* and *Aspergillus* fungi.

gastritis. Inflammation of the stomach.

gastrointestinal. Refers to the stomach and intestines.

gonad. Gland of the testis or ovary.

graft. Tissue taken from one person (donor) and transferred to another person (host).

graft-versus-host disease. A condition that can occur following an allogeneic BMT in which some of the donor's bone marrow cells (graft) attack the patient's (host's) tissues and organs. Symptoms may range from a minor skin rash to more serious complications resulting in life-threatening conditions.

granulocyte. A subclass of white blood cells, so named because of the presence of granules in the cells. These cells protect the body against bacterial infections.

hematocrit.   The percentage of the blood made up of red blood cells.

hematologist.   A doctor who specializes in the diagnosis and treatment of diseases of the blood and blood-forming tissues.

hematology.   The study of blood and its disorders.

hemoglobin.   The part of red blood cells that carries oxygen to tissues.

hemorrhage.   Bleeding.

hepatitis.   Inflammation of the liver due to a virus or toxic origin causing fever and jaundice.

Hickman catheter.   A catheter that has one end of the tubing in the heart and the other end outside the body.

host.   The person who receives the bone marrow during a bone marrow transplantation.

human leukocyte antigens (HLAs).   Proteins on the surface of cells which are important to transplantation and transfusion. For bone marrow transplants, HLAs on white blood cells are compared and only a perfect match is found with identical twins.

hyperalimentation.   Intravenous feeding that provides patients with all essential nutrients when they are unable to feed themselves. Also called hyperal, TPN, or total parenteral nutrition.

hypertension.   High blood pressure.

hypotension.   Low blood pressure.

hypothalamus.   A portion of the brain that activates, controls, and integrates part of the nervous system, endocrine processes, and bodily functions such as temperature, sleep, and appetite.

immune system.   The body's defense network against infection and foreign particles.

immunosuppression.   A condition in which the patient's immune system is functioning at a lower than normal level.

induction phase.   First phase of chemotherapy in which several powerful drugs are given to kill as many cancer cells as possible.

infiltrates.   To move into the tissue.

infusion pump.   A small, computerized device that delivers measured amounts of a drug through injection from an IV or catheter over a period of time.

inguinal nodes.   A lymph node in the upper thigh.

intensified phase.   The second phase of chemotherapy for leukemia.

intramuscular.   Injected into the muscle.

intrathecal.   Within the spinal column.   Intrathecal chemotherapy is injected into the spinal fluid.

intravenous.   Through a vein.

jaundice.   Yellowing of the skin and eyes. A sign that the liver is not functioning properly.

laminar air flow unit.   An air-filtering system used at some transplant facilities to remove particulate matter and fungi from the air.

L-asparaginase.   Chemotherapy drug used for leukemia. Must drink extra fluids to prevent kidney and bladder problems. Side effects: difficulty breathing, joint pain, skin rash, fever, abdominal pain, nausea, chills, vomiting, jaundice, confusion, drowsiness, mental depression, nervousness, swelling, sores in the mouth, severe headaches, frequent urination, unusual thirst, hallucinations, convulsions.

leukemia.   Disease of abnormal white blood cells in the bone marrow, sometimes in the spleen and liver; cancerous cells usually appear in peripheral blood and can attack other organs.

leukocyte.   White blood cell.

leukopenia.   Below-normal number of white blood cells.

lymph.   Clear, colorless fluid found in lymph vessels that carries cells to fight infection.

lymph nodes.   Oval bodies of lymphatic tissues that consist of closely packed white blood cells, connective tissue, and lymph pathways. Most lymph nodes are found in the mouth, neck, lower arm, armpit, and groin.

lymph system.   System of vessels and nodes throughout the body which helps to filter out bacteria but has other functions as well.

lymphocyte.   A type of white blood cell that helps protect the body against invading organisms by producing antibodies and regulating the immune system response. White blood cells critical to the immune system's defense against disease including cancer cells. Also known as lymphoblast.

lymphosarcoma.   A cancer of the blood-forming tissue with more bone marrow and lymph node involvement. Indistinguishable from ALL when there are more than 25% malignant cells in the marrow and it is treated exactly the same as ALL.

macrophage.   A type of white blood cell that assists in the body's fight against bacteria and infection by engulfing and destroying invading organisms.

maintenance phase.   The third or last phase of chemotherapy for leukemia. It follows the intensive induction and consolidation phases and it helps destroy any remaining cancer cells. Usually is the longest phase of treatment.

malaise.   A vague feeling of body weakness or discomfort, often indicating the beginning of disease.

methotrexate.   A chemotherapy drug to treat leukemia. Usually injected into spinal fluid for the central nervous system. Side effects: sensitivity to light, bleeding, diarrhea, sores of the mouth, abdominal pain.

monocyte.   A type of white blood cell that assists in the fight against bacteria and fungi that invade the body.

morbidity.   Sickness; side effects and symptoms of a treatment or disease.

MRI (Magnetic resonance imaging).   A method of taking pictures of body tissue using magnetic fields and radio waves.

mucositis.   Mouth sores.

myelin.   A protective covering that is like a fatty substance (for example, around the brain). Covers nerve cells.

neuro-.   Pertaining to the nervous system.

neurotoxicity.   Poisonous to nerve cells, the brain, and spinal cord.

neutropenia.   A deficiency of neutrophils (infection-fighting white blood cell).

neutrophil.   A type of white blood cell that is the body's primary defense against harmful bacteria. They ingest and destroy bacteria.

NPO.   Do not take anything by mouth.

oncologist.   A doctor who specializes in the treatment of cancer.

oncology.   Branch of medicine that studies cancer.

palliative.   Provides relief.

pancreas.   A gland behind the stomach that secretes enzymes into the intestines to aid in the digestion of food and secretes insulin for regulating carbohydrate metabolism by controlling blood sugar levels.

pancreatitis.   Inflammation of the pancreas causing pain, vomiting, hiccoughing, constipation, and collapse.

pancytopenia.   A deficiency of all types of blood cells.

pathologist.   A doctor who specializes in examining tissue to diagnose diseases.

-pathy.   Disease.

pediatrician.   A doctor who specializes in the care and development of children and the treatment of diseases.

Pediatric Oncology Group.   Organization that designs and monitors pediatric clinical trials.

-penia.   Deficiency.

peripheral blood cells.   Stem cells that circulate in the blood.

peripheral blood stem cell transplant.   Stem cells are removed from the blood, and returned after high doses of chemotherapy. This can be used for both autologous and allogeneic transplants.

peripheral neuropathy.   Injury to the nerves that supply sensation to the arms and legs.

petechiae.   Small red spots on the skin that usually indicate a low platelet count.

phlebitis.   Inflammation of a vein.

plasma.   The fluid and protein-containing portion of the blood.

platelets.   Blood cells that seal off injuries and prevent excessive bleeding without clotting.

polycythemia.   An increase in the total number of red blood cells in the bloodstream.

port-a-cath.   Catheter under the skin of the chest attached to tubing that goes to the heart.

prednisone.   A drug used during chemotherapy for leukemia to treat severe inflammation and to stop the body from having an allergic reaction. Side effects: blurred vision, frequent urination, increased thirst, skin rash, bleeding, moon face, depression, mood or mental changes, muscle cramps, pain, weakness, nausea, vomiting, stomach pain, headaches, shortness of breath, fever, tiredness.

preparative regimen.   The chemotherapy and/or radiation given to BMT patients prior to transplant to kill diseased cells and/or make space for healthy new marrow and/or suppress the immune system so graft rejection does not occur.

prognosis.   The predicted or likely outcome.

prophylactic.   Something that keeps a disease, like chemotherapy, from spreading.

protocol.   The plan of treatment.

psychopathology.   A person who exhibits an unstable mental state.

pulmonary.   Pertaining to the lungs.

purging.   Process by which certain types of cells are removed from bone marrow prior to infusion into the BMT patient. In autologous BMTs, marrow may be purged to remove lingering cancerous cells. In allogeneic BMTs, donor bone marrow may be purged to remove cells that cause graft-versus-host disease.

qualitative research.   Studies that are characterized by the use of data that is concerned with meaning or the quality and depth of participants' answers as opposed to the collection of numerical data that defines and distinguishes groups of participants.

quantitative research.   Studies that are characterized by the use of numerical data that is collected to describe or distinguish among groups of participants.

Rad.   Radiation absorbed dose.

radiation.   High-energy rays used to kill or damage cancer cells.

radiologist.   Doctor who specializes in using radiation to diagnose and treat disease.

red blood cells.   Cells that pick up oxygen from the lungs and transport it to tissues in the body.

relapse.   Recurrence of the disease following treatment.

remission, complete.   A condition in which no cancerous cells can be detected by microscope, and the patient appears to be disease-free.

remission, partial.   Generally means that by all methods used to measure the existence of a tumor, there has been at least a 50% regression of the disease following treatment.

renal.   Pertaining to the kidney.

right atrial catheter.   Catheter with tubing extending into the heart providing access for drawing blood and injecting medication.

scoliosis.   Spine curvature; sideways curve of the spine that results in an S shape of the back.

sepsis.   The presence of organisms in the blood.

side effect.   Any reaction that occurs from medication or therapy.

6-MP.   A combination chemotherapy drug melphalan plus prednisone used for leukemia. Side effects: fever, chills, sore throat, bleeding, bruising, sores in mouth and on lips, swelling, stomach pain.

somatic.   The body as distinguished from the mind.

somnolence syndrome.   Can occur 3 to 12 weeks after cranial radiation. Causes drowsiness, long periods of sleep, low-grade fever, headaches, nausea, vomiting, irritability, problems swallowing, and problems speaking.

spinal tap.   A needle is inserted at the base of the spine to extract spinal fluid to test if leukemic cells have infiltrated the central nervous system.

stem cell.   "Mother" blood cells from which several different types of blood cells evolve.

sternum (sternal).   Long flat bone in the middle of the rib cage; the breast bone.

steroid. In bone marrow transplantation, a drug commonly used in combination with other drugs to prevent and control graft-versus-host disease.

stomatitis.   Mouth sores.

stroke.   Blood clot or bleeding in the brain that causes a loss of consciousness and paralysis. Can cause injury or death to brain tissue.

syngeneic bone marrow transplant.   Transplant in which an identical twin is the bone marrow donor.

systemic. Relating to the whole body rather than to a single part.

T-cell. A type of white blood cell that can distinguish which cells belong in a person's body and which do not.

testicular morphology. Testes take on a different form and structure such as atrophy.

thrombocytes. Platelets.

total parenteral nutrition. Intravenous feeding that provides patients with all essential nutrients when they are unable to feed themselves. Also called TPN, hyperalimentation, or hyperal.

toxin. Poison.

trauma. Injury.

umbilical cord stem cells. Cord blood for transplantation is obtained at birth at no risk to mother or baby. May be frozen and stored.

veno-occlusive disease. A disease that sometimes occurs following high-dose chemotherapy and/or radiation, in which the blood vessels that carry blood through the liver become swollen and clogged.

vincrinstine. A drug that prevents the growth of cancer cells especially leukemia. Side effects: blurred vision, constipation, difficulty walking, headache, jaw and abdominal pain, joint pain, numbness in fingers and toes, pain in fingers and toes, pain in testicles, stomach cramps, weakness, agitation, bed-wetting, dizziness, convulsions, hallucinations, depression, painful urination, cough, fever, chills, shortness of breath, hair loss, bleeding, weight loss, skin rash, trouble sleeping.

virus. A tiny parasite-like agent that invades organisms, such as human cells, and alters their genetic machinery, turning them into factories for production of more of the virus.

white blood cell (WBC). Cells that help fight infection and disease (leukocytes).

whole blood. Blood that has not been separated into its various components.

xerostomia. Dryness of the mouth caused by malfunctioning salivary glands.

Appendix 3

Understanding Blood Tests

COMPLETE BLOOD COUNT (CBC)

A CBC describes the number, type, and form of each blood cell. It includes all tests described below.

RED BLOOD CELL COUNT (RBC)

Counts the number of red blood cells in a single drop (microliter) of blood. "Normal" ranges vary according to age and sex:

> Men: 4.5 to 6.2 million
> Women: 4.2 to 5.4 million
> Children: 4.6 to 4.8 million

A low RBC count may indicate anemia, excess body fluid, or hemorrhaging. A high RBC count may indicate polycythemia (an excessive number of red blood cells in the blood) or dehydration.

*Adapted with permission of S. K. Stewart (1992). *Bone marrow transplants*. Highland Park, IL: BMT Newsletter, pp. 137–139.

TOTAL HEMOGLOBIN CONCENTRATION

Hemoglobin gives red blood cells their color and carries oxygen from the lungs to cells. This test measures the grams of hemoglobin in a deciliter (100 ml) of blood, which can help physicians determine the severity of anemia or polycythemia. Normal values are:

> Men: 14 to 18 g/dl
> Women: 12 to 16 g/dl
> Children: 11 to 13 g/dl

A significant anemia occurs when the hemoglobin drops below 10 g/dl.

HEMATOCRIT

A hematocrit measures the percentage of red blood cells in the sample. Normal values vary greatly:

> Men: 45% to 57%
> Women: 37% to 47%
> Children: 36% to 40%

ERYTHROCYTE (RBC) INDICES

Three indices that measure the size of red blood cells and amount of hemoglobin contained in each:

Mean Corpuscular Volume measures the volume of red blood cells. Normal is 84 to 99 fl.

Mean Corpuscular Hemoglobin measures the amount of hemoglobin in an average cell. Normal is 26 to 32 pg.

Mean Corpuscular Hemoglobin Concentration measures the concentration of hemoglobin in red blood cells. Normal is 30% to 36%.

WHITE BLOOD CELL COUNT (WBC)

Measures the number of white blood cells in a drop (microliter) of blood. Normal values range from 4,100 to 10,900 but can be altered greatly by factors such as exercise, stress, and disease. A low WBC may indicate viral infection or toxic reactions. A high WBC may indicate infection, leukemia, or tissue damage. An increased risk of infection occurs once the WBC drops below 1,000/ml.

WBC DIFFERENTIAL

Determines the percentage of each type of white blood cell in the sample. Multiplying the percentage by the total count of white blood cells indicates the actual number of each type of white blood cell in the sample. Normal values are:

Type	Percentage	Number
Neutrophil	50–60%	3,000–7,000
Eosinophils	1–4%	50–400
Basophils	0.5–2%	25–100
Lymphocytes	20–40%	1,000–4,000
Monocytes	2–9%	100–600

A serious infection can develop once the total neutrophil count (percent of neutrophils times total WBC) drops below 500/ml.

PLATELET COUNT

Measures the number of platelets in a drop (microliter) of blood. Platelet counts increase during strenuous activity and in certain conditions called "myeloproliferative disorders": infections, inflammations, malignancies, and when the spleen has been removed. Platelet counts decrease just before menstruation. Normal values range from 150,000 to 400,000 per microliter. A count below 50,000 can result in spontaneous bleeding; below 5,000, patients are at risk of severe life-threatening bleeding.

Appendix 4

Useful Resources on Pediatric Cancer

ALL-KIDS List (Acute Lymphoblastic Leukemia)

Electronic discussion list about ALL in children. To subscribe, visit www.acor.org and click on Mailing Lists; then click on "Full listing of ACOR's public mailing lists". Scroll down to ALL-KIDS. Click on it and follow the instructions for subscribing.

Candlelighters Childhood Cancer Foundation
PO Box 498
Kensington, MD 20895-0498
Phone: 800-366-2223; 301-962-3520
Fax: 301-962-3521
E-mail: info@candlelighters.org
Web site: www.Candlelighters.org

Publications, support groups.

CaringKids

E-mail discussion list for kids who know someone who is ill. To subscribe, send an e-mail to: listserv@maelstrom.stjohns.edu. Leave subject blank (or put a dash, if subject is required). In the message, write: subscribe CaringKids and then your first and last name.

CaringParents

Electronic discussion list for adults to discuss ways to help children cope with illness (their own illness, or someone they care about). To subscribe, send an e-mail to listserv@maelstrom.stjohns.edu. Leave subject blank (or put a dash, if subject is required). In the message write: subscribe CaringParents and then your first and last name.

Children's Cancer Association (CCA)
7524 SW Macadam, Suite B
Portland, OR 97219
Phone: 503-244-3141
Fax: 503-892-1922
E-mail: office@e-cca.org
Web site: www.childrenscancerassociation.org

Information and support for children with cancer, their families and medical professionals who care for them. Programs available for those in Oregon and southwest Washington; Web site available to all.

Children's Hopes & Dreams-Wish Fulfillment Foundation
280 Route 46
Dover, NJ 07801
Phone: 800-437-3262 973-361-7366
Fax: 908-459-6627
E-mail: CHDFdover@juno.com
Web site: www.childrenswishes.org

Pen pal program for children ages 5–17, who have been diagnosed with any chronic or life-threatening illness, disability, or condition.

Children's Hospice International (CHI)
Web site: www.chionline.org

Provides a continuum of interdisciplinary care from the time of a child's diagnosis of a life-threatening condition with hope for a cure, through bereavement if cure is not attained.

Famous Fone Friends
Phone: 310-204-5683
E-mail: fonefriends@aol.com
Web site: www.nancycartwright.com/volunteer_fff.html

Celebrities telephone children who are hospitalized or homebound due to serious illness or injury. Hospitals initiate contact by providing the name and age of the child, brief medical description, phone numbers, and, sometimes, requests for specific celebrities.

Jeffrey Katz Bone Marrow Transplant Fund for Children
Los Angeles Ronald McDonald House
4560 Fountain Avenue
Los Angeles, CA 90029
Phone: 323-666-6400
Fax: 323-669-0552

Financial aid for children transplanted at UCLA.

Kids Cancer Network
PO Box 4545
Santa Barbara, CA 93140
E-mail: info@kidscancernetwork.org
Web site: www.kidscancernetwork.org

Web site with resources for children with cancer.

Kids Konnected
Phone: 800-899-2866
E-mail: info@kidskonnected.org
Web site: www.kidskonnected.org

Web site provides information and support to children who have a parent with cancer, including a chat room for kids. Adults should preview site for age appropriateness.

MEDLINEplus
Web site: medlineplus.gov

Comprehensive Web site sponsored by the National Institutes of Health that includes more than 560 health topic pages, 150 interactive slide shows, drug information, health news, medical dictionaries, and more. Also available in Spanish.

National Children's Cancer Society
1015 Locust, Suite 600
St Louis, MO 63101
Phone: 800-532-6459; 314-241-1600
Fax: 314-241-6949
E-mail: PFS@children-cancer.org
Web site: www.children-cancer.org

Financial aid, fundraising help.

Neuroblastoma Children's Cancer Society
P.O. Box 957672
Hoffman Estates, IL 60195
Phone: 800-532-5162; 847-490-4240
Fax: 847-490-0705
E-mail: info@neuroblastomacancer.org
Web site: www.neuroblastomacancer.org

Publications, emotional support.

Never-Ending Squirrel Tale
Web site: www.squirreltales.com

Web site offers tips, support, and resources for parents of children with cancer.

Pediatric Oncology Resource Center
Web site: www.acor.org/ped-onc

A Web site by and for families of children with cancer.

Pediatric-Pain
Web site: is.dal.ca/~pedpain/pedpain.html

Information on measuring and managing pain experienced by children. Easy-to-understand information can be obtained on Web site by selecting

"Self Help". Information for health care professionals also available. Created by Dalhousie University/IWK Health Centre in Nova Scotia, Canada.

PED-ONC
Web site: www.acor.org

Online support group for parents of children diagnosed with cancer. To subscribe, visit www.acor.org and click on Mailing Lists; then click on "Full listing of ACOR's public mailing lists". Scroll down to PED-ONC. Click on it and follow instructions for subscribing.

SICKKIDS Discussion List
E-mail: CaringKids-Request@maelstrom.stjohns.edu

An electronic discussion list for children (18 and under) who are ill. It is a place for kids to talk about their feelings and frustrations. To subscribe, send an e-mail to: listserv@maelstrom.stjohns.edu. Leave subject blank (or put a dash, if subject is required). In the message, write: subscribe SickKids and then your first and last name.

SuperSibs!
1566 W Algonquin Road, Suite 224
Hoffman Estates, IL 60195
Phone: 866-444-7427; toll-free 847-705-7427
Fax: 847-776-7084
E-mail: info@supersibs.org
Web site: www.supersibs.org

Free age-appropriate support for 4- to 18-year-old siblings of young cancer patients, including journals, trophies, mail, and events. Written guides are available for siblings and others for adults. In 2003, services available in the Chicagoland and Milwaukee areas; elsewhere in United States, beginning in 2004.

Appendix 5

Resource Listing Bone Marrow/Stem Cell Transplant

Information and Support

Antilogous Blood and Marrow
  Transplant
Registry (ABMTR)
  IBMTR/ABMTR Statistical
Center, Medical College of
  Wisconsin
8701 Watertown Plant Road
P.O. Box 26509
Milwaukee, WI 53226
414-456-8325
Web site: http://www.bmtsupport.
  ie/

**Blood and Marrow Transplant
Information Network**
2900 Skokie Valley Road, Suite B
Highland Park, Il 60035
888-597-7674 or 847-433-3313

The Bone Marrow Foundation
337 E. 88th St., Suite 1B

New York, NY 10128
800-365-1336 or 212-838-3029
Web site: http://www.bone
  marrow.org

**National Bone Marrow
Transplant Line (nbmtLink)**
20144 West 12 Mile Road, Suite
  108
Southfield, MI 48076
800-LINK-BMT (800-546-5268)
or 248-358-1886
Web site: http://www.nbmtlink.
  org/rg.asp

Oncology Nursing Society
125 Enterprise Drive
Pittsburgh, PA 15275
412-859-6100
Web site: http://www.ons.
  org/

Bone Marrow Donor Information

Asians for Miracle Marrow Matches
231 E. Third St., Suite 107
Los Angeles, CA 90013
888-A3M-HOPE (888-236-4673)
Web site: http::/ /www.asian_
  marrow.org/htm/getinvolvd/

Caitlin Raymond International Registry
U Mass Memorial Medical Center
55 Lake Avenue North
Worcester, MA 01655
800-766-2824 or 508-334-8969
Web site: http://www.crir.org/
  index.html

HLA Registry Foundation, Inc.
70 Grand Avenue, Suite 103

River Edge, NJ 07661
888-HLA-DONOR or 201-487-0883
Web site: http://www.holtintl.org/
  marrowtest.html

National Marrow Donor Program (NMDP)
3001 Broadway, NE Suite 500
Minneapolis, MN 55413
800-MARROW-2 or 800-526-7809
888-999-6743 (Office of Patient
  Advocacy)
Web site: http://www.marrow.org/

Orchid Diagnostic
(formerly GeneScreen)
550 West Avenue
Stamford, CT 06902
800-543-3263

Cancer Information Support

American Cancer Society
1599 Clifton Road, NE
Atlanta, GA 30329
800-ACS-2345 or 404-320-3333
Web site: http://www.cancer.org/
  docroot/home/index.asp

R.A. Bloch Cancer Foundation
4400 Main Street
Kansas City, MO 64111
800-433-0464 or 816-932-8453
Web site: http://www.blochcancer.
  org/

Cancer Care, Inc.
275 Seventh Avenue
New York, NY 10001
800-813-HOPE or 212-712-8080
Web site: www.cancercare.org

Cancer Information Service
National Cancer Institute
6116 Executive Blvd., MSC 8322
Room 3036A
Bethesda, MD 20892
800-4-CANCER
Web site: http://cis.nci.nih.gov/

Cancervive, Inc.
11635 Chayote Street
Los Angeles, CA 90049
800-426-2873 or 310-203-9232
Email: cancervivr @aol.com
www.cancervive.gov

Candlelighters Childhood Cancer Foundation
P.O. Box 498
Kensington, MD 20895
800-366-2223 or 301-962-3520
Email: info@candlelighters.org

Coping with Cancer Magazine
P.O. Box 682268
Franklin, TN 37068615-790-2400
Web site: http://www.copingmag.
  com

Cure Magazine
Cancer Information Group
3535 Worth St., Suite 4802
Dallas, TX 75246
214-820-4754
Email: editor@curetoday. com
P.O. Box 114

Friends' Health Connection
New Brunswick, NJ 08903
800-48-FRIEND or 732-418-1811

Gilda's Club Worldwide
322 Eighth Avenue, Suite 1402
New York, NY 10001
888-445-9248
Web site: http://www.gildasclub.
  org/

National Childhood Cancer Foundation
440 E. Hungtington Dr., Suite 300

Arcadia, CA 91066
800-458-6223 or 626-447-1674

National Children's Cancer Society
1015 Locust, Suite 600
St. Louis, MO 63101
800-532-6459
Web site: http://www.national
  childrenscancersociety.com

National Coalition for Cancer Survivorship
1010 Wayne Ave., Suite 770
Silver Springs, MD 20910
877-NCCS-YES or 301-650-9127
Web site: http://www.cancer
  advocacy.org

National Family Caregivers Association
10400 Connecticut Ave., Suite 500
Kensington, MD 20895
800-896-3650
Web site: http://www.starbright.
  org/

Starbright Foundation
11835 W. Olympic Blvd. Suite 500
Los Angeles, CA 90064
800-315-2580 or 310-479-1212
Web site: http://www.starbright.
  org/

Vital Options International
TeleSupport Cancer Network
15821 Ventura Blvd., Suite 645
Encino, CA 91436
818-788-5225 or 800-477-7666
Web site: http://www.personalmd.
  com/news/no717020323.shtml

Well Spouse Foundation
P.O. Box 30093
Elkins Park, PA 19027
800-838-0879
Web site: http://www.wellspouse.
  org/

The Wellness Community
35 E. Seventh St., Suite 412
Cincinnati, OH 45202
888-793-9355
Web site: http://www.wellness
  community.org/

Women's Cancer Resource Center
5741 Telegraph
Oakland, CA 94609
888-421-7900 or 510-420-7900
Web site: http://www.givingvoice.
  org/

Fertility
American Association of Tissue
  Banks
1350 Beverly Rd., Suite 220-A

McLean, VA 22101
703-827-9582
Web site: http://www.bioreposi
  tories.com

**American Society for Reproductive
  Medicine**
1209 Montgomery Highway
Birmingham, AL 35216
205-978-5000
Web site: http://www.infertility
  professionals.com/clinical/asrm.
  html

Genetics and IVF Institute
3020 Javier Road
Fairfax, VA 22031
800-552-4363 or 703-698-7355
Web site: http://www.givf.com/

Resolve, Inc.
1310 Broadway
Somerville, MA 02144
888-623-0744
Web site: http://www.resolve.org

Financial Assistance, Fundraising & Insurance Information

Cancer Legal Resource Center
919 S. Albany St.
Los Angeles, CA 90015
213-736-1455
Web site: http://www.ucdmc.
  ucdavis.edu

**Children's Organ Transplant
  Association (COTA)**
2501 COTA Drive
Bloomington, IN 47403

800-366-2682
Web site: http://www.cota.
  org

**Health Insurance Association
  of America**
1201 F. Street, NW, Suite 500
Washington, DC 20004
202-824-1600
Web site: http://www.newsin
  formers.com

Jeffrey Katz Fund
(Southern California residents)
c/o Ronald McDonald House
4560 Fountain Avenue
Los Angeles, CA 90029
323-644-3000
Web site: http://www.katzfund.
    org

The Medicine Program
P.O. Box 515
Doniphan, MO 63935
573-996-7300
Web site: http:www.freemedicine
    program.com

**My Friends Care Bone Marrow
Transplant Fund**
(Michigan residents)
148 South Main Street, Suite 101
Mount Clemens, MI 48043
586-783-7390
Web site: http://www.myfriend
    scare.org

**National Association of Hospital
Hospitality Houses**
P.O. Box 18087
Asheville, NC 28814
Web site: http://www.eparent.
    com/resources/associations/
    home_that_help.htm

**National Foundation for
    Transplants**
1102 Brookfield, Suite 200
Memphis, TN 38119
800-489-3863 or 901-684-1697
Web site: http://www.transplants.
    org

**Nielsen Organ Transplant
    Foundation**
(Northeast Florida residents)
580 West 8th St.
Jacksonville, FL 32209
888-749-4850 or 904-244-9823

**National Transplant Assistance
    Fund**
3475 West Chester Pike, Suite
    320
Newton Square, PA 19073
800-642-8399 or 610-353-9684
Web site: http://www.geocities.
    com

**Patient Advocacy Coalition,
    Inc.**
777 E. Girard Ave.
Englewood, CO 80110
303-744-7667
Web site: http://www.patient
    advocacy.net

Patient Advocate Foundation
753 Thimble Shoals Blvd. Suite
    B
Newport News, VA 23606
800-532-5274
Web site: http://www.patient
    advocate.org/

**Pharmaceutical Research and
Manufacturers of America**
Prescription Drug Patient
Assistance Programs
1100 Fifteenth St. N.W.
Washington, DC 20005
202-835-3400

Disease-Related Information

Anemia

**Aplastic Anemia & MDS
International Foundation, Inc.**
P.O. Box 613
Annapolis, MD 21404
800-747-2820 or 410-867-0242
Web site: http://www.aplastic.org

**Fanconi Anemia Research
Fund.**
1801 Williamette St. Suite 200
Eugene, OR 97401
541-687-4658
Web site: http://www.fanconi.org/

**Myeloproliferative Disease
Research Center**
115 E. 72nd St.
New York, NY 10021
800-HELP-MPD or 212-535-4200

Brain Tumor

**American Brain Tumor
Association**
2720 River Road, Suite 146
Des Plaines, IL 60018
800-886-2282 or 847-827-9910
Web site: http://www.abta.org/

**National Brain Tumor
Foundation**
414 Thirteenth St., Suite 700
Oakland, CA 94612
800-934-CURE or 510-839-9777
Web site: http://www.braintumor.
org/

Immune Deficiency Disorders

**Immune Deficiency
Foundation**
40 W. Chesapeake Ave., Suite
308
Towson, MD 21204
800-296-4433
Web site: http://www.primary
immune.org/

**National Organization for
Rare Disorders (NORD)**
P.O. Box 1968
Danbury, CT 06813
800-999-6673 or 203-744-0100
Web site: orphan@rarediseases.
Org

Leukemia & Lymphoma

**Children's Leukemia
Foundation of Michigan**
29777 Telegraph Rd., Suite
1651
Southfield, MI 48034
800-825-2536 or 248-353-8222
Email: lukemiamichigan@voyagr.
net

**The Leukemia & Lymphoma
Society**
1311 Mamoraeneck Avenue
White Plains, NY 10605
800-955-4572 or 914-949-5213
Email: infocenetr @leukemia-
lymphoma.org

Leukemia Research Foundation
(Illinois residents and those within
a 100 mile radius of Chicago)
820 Davis Street, Suite 420
Evanston, IL 60201
847-424-0600
Web site: http://www.leukemia-
    research.org

**Lymphoma Research
    Foundation
(Formerly Cure for Lymphoma)**
8800 Venice Blvd., Suite 207
Los Angeles, CA 90034
800-500-9976 or 310-204-7040
or
111 Broadway, 19th Floor
New York, NY 10006
800-235-6848 or 212-349-2910
Web site: http://www.
    lymphomaorg.healthology.
    com

**National Leukemia Research
    Association**
535 Stewart Avenue, Suite 18
Garden City, NY 11530
516-222-1944
Web site: http://www.childrens
    leukemia.org/

Multiple Myeloma

**International Myeloma
    Foundation**
12650 Riverside Drive, Suite
    206
North Hollywood, CA 91607
800-452-2873
Web site: http://www.myeloma.org

**Multiple Myeloma Research
    Foundation**
3 Forest Street
New Canaan, CT 06840
203-972-1250
Web site: http://www.multiple
    myeloma.org/

Transportation

Air Care Alliance
1515 E. 71st St. Suite 312
Tulsa, OK 74136
888-260-9707 or 918-745-0384
Web site: http://www.aircareall.
    org/

AirLifeLine
50 Fullerton Ct., Suite
    200
Sacramento, CA 95825
877-AIRLIFE or 916-641-7800
Web site: http://www.med.umich.
    edu

Corporate Angel Network
Westchester County Airport
One Loop Road
White Plains, NY 10604
866-328-1313 or 914-328-1313
Web site: http://www.corpangel
    network.org/

**National Patient Travel
    Center**
4620 Haygood Rd., Suite 1
Virginia Beach, VA 23455
800-296-1217 or 757-318-9174
Web site: http://www.npath.
    org

Information on the Internet
The Internet is a valuable tool
for cancer or medical research.
It offers a wealth of information
some helpful, some misleading.
Rely on credible sources for
information like hospitals or
medical associations. Proceed
with caution when searching on
the Internet.
Evaluate material by asking:
- What is the source of this information?
- Is it factual or opinion?
- Is it based on someone's experience?
- How current is this information?

- Is this site set up to promote a product?
When evaluating Internet sites, check the address (URL). The final segment of the address
Offers a general idea of who is sponsoring the Web site. Examples include:
.edu (site sponsored by a university)
.gov (site sponsored by a government agency)
.org (site sponsored by a nonprofit organization)
.com (site sponsored by a commercial company)

Cancer Web Site

American Society of Clinical Oncology

Breast Cancer Answers

www/camceramswers/prg

Guide to Internet Resources for Cancer

Leukemia Links

MEDLINEplus

Oncolink

ww.oncolink.org

Physicians Data Query (PDQ)

Clinical Trials Websites

clinical.html

Additional Web Sites and

Mailing Lists

AA-MDS-TALK
Listerv based mailing list in support
Of Aplastic Anemia and
Myelodysplastic Syndrome
Patients, families, and are
Providers

Association of Cancer Online Resouces (ACOR)

Offers information and support
Mailing lists about many types of
Cancer and related disorders

BMTnet
Portal to BMT resources,
Sponsored by seven International
Blood and marrow transplant
Organizations

BMT Support Online
Interactive chat for bone marrow
Transplant patients

BMT-TALK
Online communication forum

bmt-talk.html

**Bloom and Marrow Transplant
Information Network**
Lists an online database of over
250 transplant centers in the U.S.
and Canada

Health Insurance Information

**National Center for
Complementary and Alternative
Medicine**
Offers information about
Complementary medicine used in
Conjunction with standard
Treatments

Needy Meds
Information source for patient
Assistance programs

Books

**Across the Chasm, A. Caregiver's
Story** by Naomi L. Zikmund-Fisher
(BMT Infonet)

**Adult Leukemia: A Comprehen-
sive Guide for Patients And Families** by Barbara Lackritz

**Anatomy of an Illness as
Perceived by the Patient:
Reflections on Healing and
Regeneration** by Normal Coursins

**A Resource Guide for Bone
Marrow/Stem Cell Transplant**
(nbmtLink)

**Autologous Stem Cell Transplant:
A Handbook for Patients** by Sue
Stewart (BMT Infonet)

**Bone Marrow Transplants A Book
Of Basics for Patients** by
Sue Stewart (BMT Infonet)

**Cancer As a Turning Point: A
Handbook For People with Can-
cer, Their Families And Health
Professionals** by Lawrence LeShan

Cancer Talk by Selma Schimmel

**Cancer Recovery Eating Plan: The
Right Food to Help Fuel Your Recovery** by Daniel Nixon, M.D.

**Cancer Survivor's Nutrition and
Health Guide** by Gene Spiller,
PhD. And Bonnie Bruce DR.P.H.,
R.D.

The Caregiver's Companion by
Theola Jones

**Caregivers' Guide for Bone
Marrow/Stem Cell Transplant**
(nbmLink)

Choices in Healing by Michael Lerner

The Courage to Laugh: Humor, Hope, and Healing the Face of Death and Dying by Allen Klein

Everyone's Guide to Cancer Therapy, 3ʳᵈ Edition, Malin, Md. Dollinger, et al

Finding the Money: A Guide to Paying Your Bills by Diane Tolley

Full Catastrophe Living: Using The Wisdom of Your Body and Mind to Face Stress, Pain, and Illness by Jon Kabat-Zinn, Ph.D.

Getting Well Again by Carl O. Simonton, M.D. et al

Grace and Grit by Traya and Ken Wilbur

Guide to Stress Reduction by L. John Mason, Ph.D.

Healing into Life and Death By Stephen Levine

The Healing Power of Humor: Techniques for Getting Through Loss, Setbacks, Upsets, Disappointments, Difficulties, Trials, Tribulations and All That by Allen Klein

Healing Yourself: A Step-by-Step Program for Better Health

Through Imagery by Martin Rossman, M.D.

How to Live Between Office Visits By Bernie Siegel, M.D.

The Human Side of Cancer: Living with Hope, Coping with Uncertainty by Jimmie C. Holland, Sheldon Lewis

In the Country of Illness: Comfort and Advice for the Journey by Robert Lipsyte

Informed Decisions: the Complete Book of Cancer Diagnosis, Treatment and Recovery by Harmon J. Eyre

It's Always Something by Gilda Radner

The Journey Through Cancer: An Oncologist's Seven-Level Program for Healing and Transforming the Whole Person by Jeremy R. Geffen

Kitchen Table Wisdom: Stories That Heal by Rachel Naomi Remen

Learn to Relax: A Practical Guide to Easing Tension and Conquering Stress by Mike George

Learning to Fall: The Blessings Of an Imperfect Life by Philip Simmons

Love, Medicine and Miracles by Bernie Siegel

Making Informed Medical Decisions: Where to Look and How to Use What you Find by Nancy Oster

Minding the Body, Mending the Mind by Joan Borysenko, Ph.D.

Mom's Marijuana by Dan Shapiro

My Grandfather's Blessings by Rachel Naomi Remen

The New Cancer Survivors Living With Grace, Fighting with Spirit by Natalie Spingarn

Not Just one in Eight by Barbara Stevens

Peace, Love and Healing by Bernie Siegel

Stem Cell Transplant, A Companion Guide for Beast Cancer Patients (nbmtLink)

Sexuality and Cancer: For the Man/Woman Who Has Cancer and Their Partner (American Cancer Society)

Sexuality and Fertility after Cancer By Leslie R. Schover

Share Care-How to Organize a Group To Care for Someone Who

Is Seriously Ill By Cappy Capossela and Sheila Warnock

Supportive Cancer Care: The Complete Guide for Patients and Their Families By Ernest H., M.D. Rosenbaum, et al

Surviving Cancer Emotionally, Learning How to Heal by Roger Granet, M.D.

Survivor, Taking Control of Your Fight Against Cancer by Laura Landro

Take this Book to the Hospital With You: A Consumer Guide to Surviving Your Hospital Stay by Charles B. Inlander and Ed Weiner

Time on Fire by Evan Handler

Understanding Medical Information: A User's Guide to Informatics and Decision Making By Theresa Jordan

When a Parent Has Cancer: A Guide for Caring for Your Children by Wendy Schessel Harmpham, M.D.

Where the Buffaloes Roam by Bob Stone and Jenny Humphries

You Can Conquer Cancer by Ian Gawler

References

Adams, K. (2000, Feb. 7). *A brief history of journal therapy*. Lakewood, CO: The Center for Journal Therapy.

Advances in stem cell transplantation and factors affecting outcomes. (2003, October). *Blood and Marrow Transplant Newsletter*, [On-line], *14*(3), 1–3. Available: http://www.bmtinfonet.org/newsletters/issue62/advances.html

American Cancer Society. (2002). *Cancer facts and figures 2002*. Atlanta: National Cancer Institute.

Armstrong, F. D., Blumberg, M. J., & Toledano, S. R. (1999). Neurobehavioral issues in childhood cancer. *School Psychology Quarterly, 28,* 194–203.

Armstrong, F. D., & Horn, M. (1995). Educational issues in childhood cancer. *School Psychology Quarterly, 10,* 292–304.

Baker, J. E., Sedney, M.A., & Gross, E. (1992). Psychological tasks for bereaved children. *American Journal of Orthopsychiatry, 62,* 105–116.

Bartel, N. R., & Thurman, S. K. (1992). Medical treatment and educational problems in children. *Kappan, 74*(1), 57–61.

Beckman, R. (1990). *Children who grieve: A manual for conducting support groups.* Montreal: Learning Publications.

Berg, C. (1978). Helping children accept death and dying through group counseling. *Personnel and Guidance Journal, 57*(8), 169–172.

Candlelighters Childhood Cancer Foundation. (2003, Spring). Invitation to submit your child's artwork for network. *Quarterly Journal of the National Office.* 1–11.

Chesler, M. A., Weigers, M., & Lawther, T. (1992). How am I different? Perspectives of childhood cancer survivors on change and growth. In D. M. Green & G. D'Angio (Eds.), *Late effects of treatment for childhood cancer* (pp. 151–158). New York: Wiley.

Children's Cancer Web. (2003, January). Cancer Types: Leukemia. Available: http://www.cancerindex.org.

Chomicki, S., Sobsey, D., Sauvageot, D., & Wilgosh, L. (1995). Surviving the loss of a child with a disability: Is loss the end of chronic sorrow? *Physical Disabilities: Education and Related Services, 13*(2), 17–30.

Cognitive effects to the brain—part II. (2003, October). *Candlelighters Childhood Cancer Foundation* [On-line]. Available: http://www.candlelighters.org/treatmentcoglaeeffects1.stm

Counts, D. R., & Counts, D. A. (1991). *Coping with the final tragedy: Cultural variations in dying and grieving.* Amityville, NY: Baywood.

Crenshaw, D. A. (1990). *Bereavement: Counseling the grieving throughout the life cycle.* New York: Continuum

Dahlgren, T., & Praeger-Decker, I. (1979) A unit on death for primary grades. *Health Education, 10*(1), 36–39.

Doka, K. J. (1995). *Children mourning, mourning children.* Washington, DC: Hospice Foundation of America .

Dahlgren, T., & Prager-Decker, I. (1979) A unit on death for primary grades. *Health Education, 10*(1), 36–39.

Eddy, J. M., & Alles, W. F. (1983). *Death education.* St. Louis: C. V. Mosby.

Eiser, C., Havermans, T., & Eiser, J. (1995). Parents' attitudes about childhood cancer: Implications for relationships with medical staff. *Child Care, Health, and Development, 21*(1), 31–42.

Feifel, H. (Ed.). (1977). *New meanings of death.* New York: McGraw-Hill.

Fobair, P. (1996, Spring). National and local trends: Concern for long-term and late side effects of cancer treatment. *Surviving.*

Fredlund, D. (1977). Children and death from the school setting view point. *The Journal of School Health, 47*, 533–537.

Goodman M., Rubinstein R., Alexander B., Luborsky M., (1991). Cultural differences among elderly women coping with the death of an adult child. *Journal of Gerontology, 46*(6), 321–329.

Harper, D. C., & Wadsworth, J. S. (1993). Grief in adults with mental retardation: Preliminary findings. *Research in Developmental Disabilities, 14*, 313–330.

Helms, R., & Blazer, D. (1986). *What about the children? Dealing with death.* (ERIC Reproduction Services No. ED 193-298).

Hickey, L. O. (1993). Death of a counselor: A bereavement group for junior high school students. In N. B. Webb (Ed.), *Helping the bereaved child* (pp. 239–266). New York: Guilford Press.

Hoekstra-Weebers, J., Jaspers, J., Kamps, W., & Klip, E. (1998). Gender differences in psychological adaptation and coping in parents of pediatric cancer patients. *Psycho-Oncology, 7*, 26–36.

Holland, J. (1993). Child bereavement in Humberside primary schools. *Educational Research, 35*, 289–297.

Kandt, V. E. (1994). Adolescent bereavement: Turning a fragile time into acceptance and peace. *The School Counselor, 41*, 103–211.

Kaplan, D., Smith, A., & Grobstein, R. (1974). School management of the seriously ill child. *The Journal of School Health, 44*(5), 250–254.

Kazak, A. E. (1994). Implications of survival: Pediatric oncology patients and their families. In D. J. Bearison & R. K. Mulhern (Eds.), *Pediatric psychooncology: Psyhcological perspectives on children with cancer* (pp. 171–193).

Keene, N. (1999). In *Childhood leukemia: A guide for families, friends, caregivers* (2nd ed.). Subastopol California: O'Reilly & Associates. pp. 1–513.

Keith, C., & Ellis, D. (1978). Reactions of pupils and teachers to death in the classroom. *The School Counselor, 25*(4), 228–235.

Kelker, K., Hecimovic; A, & Leroy, C. H. (1994). Designing a classroom and school environment for students with AIDS. *Teaching Exceptional Children, 26*(4), 52–55.

Kloeppel, D. A., & Hollins, S. (1989). Double handicap: Mental retardation and death in the family. *Death Studies, 13*, 31–38.

Knowles, D., & Reeves, N. (1981). Understanding children's concerns about death and dying. B. C. *Journal of Special Education, 5*(1), 33–40.

Koocher, G. P., & O'Malley, J. E. (1981). *The Damocles syndrome: Psychological consequences of surviving childhood cancer.* New York: McGraw-Hill.

Landers, S. (2003, July). Complicated history: What happens when cancer servivors grow up? Available: http://www.ama-assn.org/amednews/2003/07/07/hlsa0707.htm (pp.1–6).

Ledoux, D. (1993). *Turning memories into memoirs: A handbook for writing life stories.* Lisbon Falls, ME: Soleil Press.

List, M., Ritter-Sterr, C., & Lansky, S. (1992). Enhancing the adjustment of long-term survivors: Early findings of a school intervention study. In D. M. Green & G. D'Angio (Eds.), *Late effects of treatment for childhood cancer* (pp. 159–164). New York: Wiley.

Madan-Swain, A., Brown, R. T., Ealco, G. A., Cherrick, I., Ievers, C. E., Conte, P. M., Vega, R., Bell, B., & Lauer, S. J. (1998, October–November). Cognitive, academic, and psychosocial late effects among children previously treated for acute lymphocytic leukemia receiving chemotherapy as CNS prophylaxis. *Journal of Pediatric Psychology, 23*, 333–340.

Marina, N. (1997). Long-term survivors of childhood cancer: The medical consequences of cure. *Pediatric Oncology, 4*(4), 1021–1042.

McDaniel, B. A. (1989). A group work experience with mentally retarded adults on the issues of death and dying. *Journal of Gerontological Social Work, 13*, 187–191.

McDougal, S. (1997, December) *Children with cancer: Side effects and educational implications* [Online], Pediatric Oncology Resource Center Web site. Available: http://www.acor.org/ped-onc/cfissues/backtoschool/cwc.html

McEvoy, J. (1989). Investigating the concept of death in adults who are mentally handicapped. *British Journal of Mental Subnormality, 35*, 115–121.

McLaughlin, T. E. (1994). Death of a leader. *The American School Board Journal, 181*(8), 40–41.

McLoughlin, I.]., & Bhate, M. S. (1987). A case of affective psychosis following bereavement in a mentally handicapped woman. *British Journal of Psychiatry, 151*, 552–554.

Memmott, C. (1995, July–September). Low-key philanthropist: Paul Newman puts his talents to use helping others. *Leadership, 27*.

Mishler, E. G. (1986). *Research interviewing*. Cambridge, MA: Harvard University Press.

Mulhern, R. K. (1994). Neuropsychological late effects. In D. J. Bearison & R. K. Mulhern (Eds.), *Pediatric psychooncology: Psychological perspectives on children with cancer* (pp. 99–121).

Mulhern, R. K., Wasserman, A. L., Friedman, A. G., & Fairclough, D. (1989). Social competence and behavioral adjustment in children who are long-term survivors of cancer. *Pediatrics, 83*, 18–25.

Munroe, R., & Munroe, R. (1975). *Cross-cultural human development*. Monterey, CA: Brooks-Cole Publishing.

Munsch, M. (1993). School-based intervention following violent death—a classmate's family. In N. B. Webb (Ed.), *Helping the bereaved child* (pp. 267–285). New York: Guilford Press.

National Cancer Institute. (2002). *Young people with cancer: A handbook for parents*. Bethesda, MD: National Institutes of Health.

National Children's Cancer Foundation. (1997). *Facts about childhood cancer* [Online]. Available: http://www.nccf.org/childhoodcancer/different.asp.

Nir, Y. (1995). Posttraumatic stress disorder in children with cancer. In S. Eth & R. Pynoos (Eds.), *Posttraumtic Stress Disorder in Children*. Washington, DC: American Psychiatric Press.

O'Brien, J. M., Goodenow, C., & Espin, O. (1991). Adolescent's reaction to the death of a peer. *Adolescence, 26*, 431–440.

Peckham, V. C. (1993). Children with cancer in the classroom. *Teaching Exceptional Children, 26*, 26–32.

Pendergast, D. E. (1995). Preparing for children who are medically fragile in education programs. *Teaching Exceptional Children, 27*(2), 37–41.

Phipps, S., Fairclough, D., & Mulhern, R. K., (1995). Avoidant coping in children with cancer. *Journal of Pediatric Psychology, 20*, 217–232.

Pickett, M. (1993). Cultural awareness in the context of terminal illness. *Cancer Nursing, 16*(2), 102–106.

Rait, D., Ostroff, J., Smith, K., Cells, D., Tan, C., & Lesko, L. (1992, December). Lives in the balance: Perceived family functioning and psychosocial adjustment of adolescent cancer survivors. *Family Process, 31*(4), 383–397.

Randall, F. (1984, January 29). Why scholars become storytellers. *New York Times Book Review*, pp. BR1, 2.

Reeves, N., & Knowles, D. (1981). Helping children deal with death concerns. B.C. *Journal of Special Education, 5*(1), 41–48.

Research findings hold promise for leukemia, blood cancer patients. (2001, April). *Bone Marrow Transplant Newsletter, 15*(2), 4.

Resource guide for bone marrow/stem cell transplant: Friends helping friends. (2001). *National Bone Marrow Transplant Link* [On-line]. Available: http://www.comnet.org/nbmtlink

Roman, D. D., & Sperduto, P. W. (1995). Neuropsychological effects of cranial irradiation: Current knowledge and future directions. *International Journal of Radiation Oncology, Biology, Physics, 31*, 983–998.

Romanoff, B. D. (1993). When a child dies: Special considerations for providing mental health counseling for bereaved parents. *Journal of Mental Health, 12*, 384–393.

Rosenthal, N. R. (1980). Death education: Help or hurt. *The Clearing House, 53*, 224–226.

Rubenstein, C. L., Varni, J. W., & Katz, E. R. (1990). Cognitive functioning in long-term survivors of leukemia: A perspective analysis. *Developmental and Behavioral Pediatrics, 11*, 301–305.

Rucker, M., Thompson, L., & Dickerson, B. (1978). Puppet life and death education. *The Clearing House, 1*, 458–459.

Sandoval, C. (2001). Acute lymphoblastic leukemia. [On-line]. Available: http://www.Mckenziebanner.healthology.com.

Sargent, J., Olle, J., Roghmann, K., Mulhern, R., Barbarian, O., Carpenter, P., Copeland, D., Dolgin, M., & Zeltzer, L. (1995). Sibling adaptation to childhood cancer collaborative study: Siblings' perceptions of the cancer experience. *Journal of Pediatric Psychology, 20*(2), 151–162.

School in session even with cancer: Learning gives pediatric patients education and hope. (2003, September). *Cancer Wise,* [On-line]. University of Texas M. D. Anderson Center. Available: http://www.cancerwise.org/

Sexson, S. B., & Madan-Swain, A. (1993). School reentry for the child with chronic illness. *Journal of Learning Disabilites, 26*, 115–125.

Smyth, J. M., Stone, A. A., Hurewitz, A., & Kaell, A. (1999, April). Effects of writing about styressful experiences on symptom reduction in patients with asthma or rheumatoid arthritis: a randomized trial. *Journal of the American Medical Association, 281*(14), 1304–9.

Snyder, T. D. (1993). When tragedy strikes: Helping students and staff cope with loss. *Executive Educator, 15*(7), 30–31.

Spice, B. (1997, February 9). Boy battles leukemia as doctors try to learn why he is succeeding. *Pittsburgh Post-Gazette*, p. C-1.

Spinelli, C. G. (2003, Spring). Educational and psychosocial implications affecting childhood cancer survivors: What educators need to know. *Physical Disabilities: Education and Related Services, 21*(2), 49–65.

Spinelli, C. G. (2004). Dealing with cancer in the classroom: The teacher's role and responsibilities. *Teaching Exceptional Children, 36*(4), 14–21.

Spinetta, J., & Deasy-Spinetta, P. (Eds.). (1981). *Living with childhood cancer.* St. Louis: C. V. Mosby.

Srikameswaran, A. (1994, July 4). Families cope with cancer in more than 1. *Pittsburgh Post-Gazette*, pp. 1, 15, 16.

Staley, L. (2000). Time to say good-bye. *Childhood Education, 76*(3), 170.

Steen, G. & Mino, J. (Eds.). (2000, April). *Childhood cancer: A handbook from St. Jude's Children's Research Hospital.* New York: Perseus.

Stuber, M., Kazak, A., Meeske, K., Barakat, L., Gutherie, D., Garnier, H., Pynoos, R., & Meadows, A. (1997, December). Predictors of posttraumatic stress symptoms in childhood cancer survivors. *Pediatrics, 100*(6), 958–964.

Sullivan, N. (1995). *Educational implications of surviving childhood acute lymphoblastic leukemia and its treatment regimes: Perspectives and reflections of long-term survivors.* Unpublished doctoral dissertation, University of Pittsburgh.

Sullivan, N., Fulmer, D., & Zigmond, N. (2000, Fall). Returning to school: Reintegration of survivors of childhood acute lymphoblastic leukemia. *Physical Disabilities: Education and Related Services, 19*(1), 25–53.

Sullivan, N., Fulmer, D., & Zigmond, N. (2001, Fall). School: The normalizing factor for children with childhood leukemia: Perspectives of young survivors and their parents. *Preventing School Failure, 46*(1), 4–13.

Tait, P. E., & Ward, P. (1987). When a student dies: Helping teachers who grieve. *Education of the Visually Handicapped, 18*, 151–156.

Thompson, S. J., Leigh, L., Christensen, R., Xiong, X., Kun, L. E., Heidman, R. L., Reddick, V. E., Gajjar, A., Merchant, T., Pui, C. H., Hudson, M. M., & Mulhern, R. K. (2001). Immediate neurocognitive effects of methylpenidate on learning-impaired survivors of childhood cancer. *Journal of Clinical Oncology, 19*(6), 1802–1808.

Thornton, C., & Krajewski, J. (1993). Death education for teachers: A refocused concern relative to medically fragile children. *Intervention in School and Clinic, 29*(1), 31–35.

Tyc, L., Mulhern, R., & Bieberich, A. (1997). Anticipatory nausea and vomiting in pediatric cancer patients: An analysis of conditioning and coping variables. *Developmental and Behavioral Pediatrics, 18*(1), 27–33.

Varni, J. W., Katz, E. R., Colegrave, R., & Dolgin, M. (1994). Perceived social support and adjustment of children with newly diagnosed cancer. *Developmental and Behavioral Pediatrics, 15,*20–26.

Wadsworth, J. S., & Harper, D. C. (1991). Grief and bereavement in mental retardation: A need for new understanding. *Death Studies, 15*, 281–292.

Webb, N. B. (1993). Assessment of the bereaved child. In N. B. Webb (Ed.), *Helping the bereaved child* (pp. 19–42). New York: Guilford Press.

Well-Connected. (2000, January). *Who gets acute lymphoblastic leukemia?* [Online], pp. 1–5. Available: http://wellness.ucdavis.edu/medical_conditions_az/alleukemia86.html.

Yapa, P., & Clarke, D. J. (1989). Schizophreniform psychosis associated with delayed grief in a man with moderate handicap. *Mental Handicap Research, 2*, 211–212.

Index

About the Author

NANCI A. SULLIVAN has 25 years of experience in education as a practitioner, researcher, and administrator. She received a B.S. degree in elementary and special education from Franciscan University of Steubenville. She attained an M.S. degree in education administration from the University of Dayton. She achieved an Ed.D. in education/special education from the University of Pittsburgh and through a postdoctoral program at Duquesne University she received the Superintendent's Letter of Eligibility. Dr. Sullivan has taught special education students in public schools, participated in research projects, presented research nationally and internationally at conferences, visited and consulted with schools in seven other countries, and she has been a public school administrator in the areas of special education and pupil personnel. She has been presented with awards for both her teaching and research abilities. She currently resides in Pittsburgh, Pennsylvania.